MW01250796

The information provided in this book is designed to provide helpful information on the subjects discussed. This book is not meant to be used, nor should it be used, to diagnose or treat any medical condition. For diagnosis or treatment of any medical problem, consult your own physician. The publisher and author are not responsible for any specific health or allergy needs that may require medical supervision and are not liable for any damages or negative consequences from any treatment, action, application or preparation, to any person reading or following the information in this book. References are provided for informational purposes only and do not constitute endorsement of any websites or other sources. Readers should be aware that the websites listed in this book may change.

WHAT THIS BOOK IS NOT!

Whilst I have referred where appropriate to important medically based studies, books and medical papers, this book has not been written as a medical research paper, designed to cover dozens of scientific subjects.

I have deliberately avoided the current trend in many diet books to constantly cherry pick medical and scientific studies to support the book's conclusions. This book is not intended as a reference item to satisfy those readers that might be looking for useful research material.

This book is about a real life journey and the real life testing processes that have identified the most effective ways to develop great eating behaviours and incorporating those behaviours into our daily food choices.

There will be a detailed bibliography attached to this book. This is a truly exciting and rapidly evolving science and there is a vast amount of material to read and study about Epigenetics, Ketogenics, Palaeolithic Eating Selection and Functional Medicine in general, especially in the way that these insights apply to intelligent weight management. If you require further information, I suggest you contact me for specific recommendations at

beranparry@gmail.com

FIGHTING FIBROMYALGIA With THE ANTI- INFLAMMATORY DIET By Mercedes Del Rey

<u>Special Free Gift from one of my friends</u>

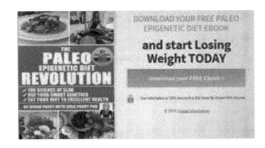

Please search for this page http://www.skinnydeliciouslife.com/free-epigenetic-diet-ebook

BY THE SAME AUTHOR

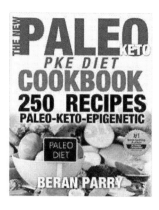

Please search this page over the internet https://www.amazon.com/s/ref=nb_sb_noss?url=search-alias%3Ddigital-text&field-keywords=B013EZAZO8

FIGHTING FIBROMYALGIA

With THE

ANTI- INFLAMMATORY

DIET

Free 21 Day Anti Inflammatory Eating Plan

By

Mercedes Del Rey

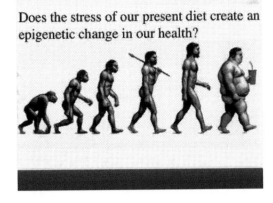

Does the stress of our present diet create an epigenetic change in our health?

FROM THE AUTHOR

So much has changed in our understanding of how the human body functions. New research, dramatic developments in how we measure what happens inside our bodies, revolutionary shifts in the way we're applying this new knowledge to help people overcome serious medical conditions.

You might still hear the occasional explanation that bad genes account for so much excess weight, disease or ill-health. It's time to put that outdated and misleading concept in the rubbish bin where it belongs. This is where the most astonishing research into human genetics has demonstrated that many of our genes are not fixed. They can be switched on and off.

That means that genetic indicators for many medical conditions can be influenced by environmental factors - and that includes the food we eat. That's right. We can no longer blame our ancestors for all of our inherited conditions. It's about lifestyle choices and putting the responsibility for our health, our weight and our wellbeing firmly back in our own hands. The PKE Dietary Revolution listens to your body and helps you to feel as amazing as your body really wants you to feel. The Revolutionary begins today!

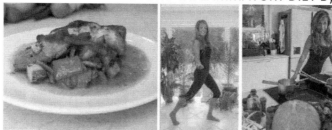

Table of Contents

Chapter 1 What is Inflammation? And how does Ketosis Help?

It is becoming increasingly clear that chronic inflammation is the root cause of many serious illnesses - including FIBROMYALGIA. We all know inflammation on the surface of the body as local redness, heat, swelling and pain. It is the cornerstone of the body's healing response, bringing more nourishment and more immune activity to a site of injury or infection. But when inflammation persists or serves no purpose, it damages the body and causes illness. Stress, lack of exercise, genetic predisposition, and exposure to toxins (like secondhand tobacco smoke) can all contribute to such chronic inflammation, but dietary choices play a big role as well. Learning how specific foods influence the inflammatory process is the best strategy for containing it and reducing long-term disease risks. (Find more details on the mechanics of the inflammation process and the Anti-Inflammatory Food Pyramid.)

Andrew Weil MD

Recently a new study was published which looked at the potential mechanisms underlying the specific anti-inflammatory properties of ketosis

For those unfamiliar, a ketogenic diet is one which contains very little – if any – carbohydrate‑   One classic example of this dietary approach is seen in the Inuit people.‑   The Inuit are indigenous people, who live in the Arctic region.

Alaska, Canada and Greenland all have Inuit populations.

In one of the more famous nutrition stories of recent times, Dr. Vilhjalmur Stefansson ate nothing but meat for one year, after being inspired by living with the Inuit, and seeing their remarkably low rate of disease

This was despite the Inuit's (then) controversial diet of nothing but meat, whether it came from fish or other sources. Stefansson saw no ill effects from a year of an all meat diet, with basically zero carbohydrate. He also consumed no vegetables. It is worth noting, that he also became very ill when he consumed only low fat meat, and nothing else. When he added the fattier meat back in, he immediately felt better.

The many reported benefits of the ketogenic diet include, but are not limited to: less hunger while dieting, improved cognitive function in those who are cognitively impaired, improved LDL cholesterol levels, improved weight loss, and improved levels of HDL_cholesterol

This is in addition to the aforementioned anti-inflammatory effects. When we look to the scientific literature, we see that the anti-inflammatory nature of the diet has been studied for many years.

The ketogenic diet has also been established as an adequate anticonvulsant therapy.

This newly published research looks specifically at the ketone metabolite beta-hydroxybutyrate, which seems to inhibit the NLRP3 inflammasome

Since the NLRP3 inflammasome was previously found to have been linked to obesity and inflammation, as well as insulin resistance, inhibiting it would make mechanistic sense.[27] The resultant weight loss and anti-inflammatory effects, commonly seem (at least anecdotally) when adopting a ketogenic diet, would then make sense as well. The NLRP3 inflammasome also drives the inflammatory response in several disorders including autoimmune diseases, type 2 diabetes, Alzheimer's disease, atherosclerosis, and auto inflammatory disorders

.

Could it all be so simple? Possibly, though there is certainly likely more to be more scientific discoveries, relating to the beneficial effects of this specific dietary approach. Moving away from glucose and instead utilizing ketone bodies as a source of metabolic fuel, results in many profound changes, of which we are only beginning to scratch the surface of, scientifically.

This new discovery will likely be the first of many new findings regarding the ketogenic diet, and its abundance of benefits. If you are looking to adopt a ketogenic approach, simply follow the Paleo Diet, and then lower your carbohydrate intake to below 100g per day.

How low you need to go for optimum quality of life is highly variant, and many people report different results with different amounts of carbohydrates.

In recent years, three excellent clinical studies have been published that utilized what the authors called a Spanish ketogenic Mediterranean diet.

The diet consisted of olive oil, moderate red wine, green vegetables and salads, fish as the primary protein, as well as lean meat, fowl, eggs, shellfish and cheese. (Nuts are also acceptable, although they were not included in these studies.) Notice that absolutely no sugar, flour, whole grains, or legumes were consumed. Fruit was also not included.

What is a Ketogenic diet?

The Ketogenic diet is a low carb, high fat diet with majority of calories provided by fat , minimal carbs and moderate protein. Contrary to the general belief the fat used in Ketogenic diet, essentially from medium chain fatty acids, are not associated with worsening heart and vascular disease. Medium chain fatty acids have a denser energy potential and is easily converted to ATP for cell consumption.

The ketogenic diet is used to manage a variety of conditions such as diabetes, metabolic syndrome, polycystic ovarian syndrome, obesity, hypertension, epilepsy, gastroesophageal reflux disease and irritable bowel syndrome.

Ketogenic diet has been used since 1920s very effectively to control refractory seizures of childhood epilepsy. It fell out of favor after the introduction of Dilantin the anti seizure medication.

What are ketones?

Ketons are produced in the body when the fats are burned. Ketons are primarily used when glucose is not readily available to be used for fuel. By adopting a Ketogenic diet your body adopts to use fat instead of carbohydrates to obtain fuel for cellular daily function.

Ketone bodies can be used for energy source for most of the normal cells. There is growing evidence that ketones have beneficial effects on aging, inflammation, metabolism, cognition and athletic performance.

Our ancestors used Ketogenic type diet during the non-animal based food shortage and it is known that new born that are strictly breast fed go into Ketogenic state and 25% of their energy needs are supplied by ketones. So nature has already adopted itself to adopt to this type of dietary habits.

The main ketones produced that are measurable in the blood or urine are beta hydroxybutyrate (blood) , acetoacetate (urine) acetone (breath).

What are the benefits of a low carb, high fat diet namely nutritional ketosis state?

1. Ketones are the preferred fuel source for liver, brain , heart and muscle.

2. Ketosis is an excellent way of losing body fat

3. By being keto-adapted you generate fuel from dietary fat and body fat but when we consume excess carbohydrate, it is turned into fat and not easily digested to fuel.

4. Natural hunger and appetite control

5. Effortless weight loss and maintenance

6. Mental clarity

7. Better sleep

8. Normalized metabolic function

9. Stabilized blood sugar and increased cellular insulin sensitivity

10. Lower inflammation in the body

11. Blood pressure control

12. Better cholesterol control with increase in good cholesterol (HDL) and decrease in bad cholesterol (LDL) and triglycerides

13. Better fertility

14. Improved immune system

15. Reduction of free radicals and slowing the aging process

16. Improve in cognitive function and memory

17. Decreased anxiety and mood swings

18. Decreased heartburn

19. Felling general well being and happiness

Let's Start

Chapter 2 What is Fibromyalgia and How do we deal with it?

Fibromyalgia is a painful and often distressing condition that mainly targets women and, despite an abundance of theories about the possible origins of this syndrome, no one knows for certain what causes it. The disease seems to increase nerve sensitivity in the spinal cord or brain and the most obvious symptom of the condition is the constant and often debilitating presence of pain. The discomfort can vary in intensity from hour to hour and from day to day. It can afflict people as young as 30 but it seems to be more common from the age of 40 to 50. The challenge for medical science lies in the fact that it is difficult to treat a condition where the causes are unknown. Despite the claims from some quarters, there is no known, medically-sanctioned cure for Fibromyalgia. Yet people have experienced degrees of relief from the pain by taking pain-killers and, perhaps more importantly, by changing their diet and lifestyle. There is some evidence that suggests that Fibromyalgia may be provoked by the effects of long-term food intolerances and this theory might explain why the syndrome tends to appear later in life as a result of several decades of accumulated intolerances.

The conventional, medical approach to Fibromyalgia is to treat the problem with prescription medication and that typically involves Cox-2 inhibitors and anti-infammatory drugs. The idea is to reduce the sufferer's hyper-sensitivity to pain, although it's important to recognise the potential for serious side-effects from the mainstream drugs that are often prescribed.

Despite the general uncertainty surrounding the causes of Fibromyalgia, sufferers still need to attend their doctors on a regular basis to keep up to date with the latest developments in treatment and drug therapy. But experimenting with diet can help people to feel that they're able to influence the condition and assume a greater degree of control over their pain. This is very important from a psychological perspective and helps individuals to regain a sense of hope that can be deeply empowering. It woud appear that when we give up and quit our efforts to contend with the problem, it's just too easy to settle into a depressing slump of dejection and create an expectation that the condition will only deteriorate further. Encouraging sufferers to remain cheerful and adopt a robust sense of humour doesn't always help to cope with the pain. We all experience pain in a deeply personal and individualistic manner and suggestions to shrug off the discomfort, though well-intentioned, aren't always helpful to the person who's in pain.

When you're diagnosed with Fibromyalgia, one of the more helpful strategies is to recognise that you're not alone. You're not the only sufferer and it can be reassuring to join a local support group, access on-line discussion groups and bulletin boards and check for developing information on the Internet. The research is not static. It's evolving every day. There's also a growing body of experience-based concensus on what constitutes a healthy diet for Fibromyalgia sufferers. It might not apply equally to everyone for the simple reason that the condition exhibits such a wide variety of symptoms but there are planty of very helpful clues that could change the pain profile of many sufferers.

It's a well established fact that food intolerances can play a significant role in exacerbating a number of inflammatory conditions so, a Fibromyalgia diet would seek to exclude certain common, potential allergens.

For example, in a study of rheumatoid arthritis patients, 91% of the sample experienced a measurable improvement in their symptoms after eliminating grains, dairy produce, nuts, beef, eggs and certain other foods from their diets. The recent research on the inflammatory effects of gluten would naturally eliminate grains from the daily diet. The widespread intolerance to the caseine that occurs in dairy products would offer another range of products for exclusion too.

But the pattern is more complex than might appear at first glance. For some individuals, symptoms have eased increasing red meat consumption whilst cutting back on wheat and dairy. Despite the apparent contradiction, it still appears that food intolerances and allergies are the main culprits. It's obvious that individuals will express their own reactions to allergies and food sensitivities, so we would expect some variety in the ways that Fibromyalgia diets are desribed for different individuals.

The easiest way to launch your own experiment to determine which specific food types may be causing a reaction, simply start by eliminating the most common types of food allergens - and that list includes grains, dairy, nuts, meat and eggs. You could also try following a Vegan Fibromyalgia diet for ten days. This will provide adequate time for your body to show any improvements. Then by simply adding grains, dairy, nuts, meat and eggs to your daily diet, one at a time, you should be able to identify any foods that have been causing you a problem. Your body becomes your very own, personal research lab and you get to confirm the results day by day.

It's significant to note that in the rheumatoid arthritis study, 86% of patients reported that certain foods repeatedly aggravated their symptoms. However, not all foods had to be eliminated from the final diet. Most people only had to eliminate two or three problem items.

In his book, Foods that Fight Pain, Dr. Neal Barnard extended the list of most common allergens by including chocolate, caffeine, citrus fruits, tomatoes, onions, corn, apples and bananas. With the exception of corn, apples and bananas, these foods are all highly acidic and may be a source of problems for people with digestive complaints, such as acid reflux.

Amongst the many ideas currently circulating about Fibromyalgia relief, some individuals claim to have obtained great results by using a product called XangoT, which is made from a Southeast Asian fruit called the mangosteen.

XangoT made from mangosteen and is now available in the United States as a puree juice blend of both the rind and the mangosteen fruit. The mangosteen rind was used historically throughout India and Asia

FIGHTING FIBROMYALGIA With THE ANTI- INFLAMMATORY DIET By Mercedes Del Rey

to treat a wide variety of painful conditions, which might explain why it is being recommended by some doctors as a source of relief from Fibromyalgia.

For example, Dr. J Frederic Templeman, M.D., states that: "Although no other intervention has ever helped even 45% of my patients, in my experience, mangosteen can brief relief, either partial or complete, to over 60% of sufferers." By sufferers, Dr. Templeman is referring to individuals afflicted with Fibromyalgia and its range of painful symptoms.

There may be a solid, scientific explanation for mangosteen's success as a pain inhibitor. Research has demonstrated that the mangosteen rind or fruit contain components which inhibit Cox-2, as well as being anti-inflammatory and anti-allergenic.

The growing number of reports supporting mangosteen's effectiveness as a pain reliever suggest that this kight be a very helpful product to add to a sufferer's daily routine.

It seems apparent from the research that oversensitive nerve cells are one of the major problems of Fibromyalgia. If the mangosteen extracts can protect nerve tissue from damage and prevent or counteract the effects of age and oxidation, they can only serve to alleviate the symptoms of many sufferers. If low blood sugar is also a problem, the mangosteen has been shown to help stabilize blood sugar levels. The Cox-2 inhibitor in mangosteen appears to be more powerful than some of the drugs that are prescribed for Fibromyalgia but, reassuringly, this exotic fruit seems to work without any of the side effects associated with prescribed pharmaceuticals.

Adapting to Work

Fibromyalgia is a progressive disease that can take up to twenty years to manifest its fullest severity. It does not appear overnight. It tends to advance slowly over time. And this gradual increase in discomfort will eventually impinge on the sufferer's ability to work. These are eminently practical issues and the sooner the situation is `ssessed, the more time you will have to plan for the future, especially if that involves quitting work, retiring early or opting for redundancy. None of these choices may be appealing but, if the condition deteriorates too far, work maighr simply become untenable. Having an alternative strategy, cutting back on expenses, moving to a more manageable property and preparing for a possible reduction in income will ease the blow of no longer being employed. There are plenty of personal issues to contend with too as women slowly lose the energy to take care of their homes and partners. It's a situation that can put a great deal of strain on any relationship. Learning to talk to each other and preserving the ability to laugh and understand one another can make a world of difference to a difficult set of circumstances.

Mobility

Even walking can be painful, running impossible, climbing stairs difficult and perhaps, eventually, you might consider moving home or installing some kind of stair lift. Driving a car may be hard, even dangerous, getting on buses a tough task, so the easy option is to spend more and more time at home.

You might become much more reliant on the Internet for shopping and get your groceries delivered to your home. A mobile phone and a computer may become your main connections to the outside world.

Sleep

Pain interferes with normal sleep, causing you to wake up during the night and change position frequently. Your mind is restless and you may go to bed deeling tired and then stay awake for hours on end. Your bed partner may join you, unwillingly, in your restless night of disturbed sleep, and this can further increase tensions between you.

Getting a better bed may make a difference or experimenting with a different bedtime schedule. If your nighttime sleep is disturbed, you ight benefit from a daytime nap to help you to recharge batteries.

Getting up in the morning may be especially hard and it can be uncomfortable since the body can feel naturally stiffer.

Caring

Fibromyalgia is rarely suffered in isolation. It affects everyone in the family constellation. Those who are charged with caring for sufferers may accept their role with pleasure or reluctance. It can be particularly tough for children who find themselves caring for their parents.

Since there are no obvious outward signs that a person is suffering from Fibromyalgia, many people may be less than sympathetic about the condition. Even in cases where the sufferer complains of pain or of having a bad day, it's often viewed by sceptics as being "all in the mind" or the sufferer is accused of exaggerating. Close family members, who often feel that they are carrying much of the burden of care, are often the worst offenders in the sympathy stakes.

Yet against this background of suffering, we need to remember that there are still grounds for hope. Experimenting with diet, re-balancing the intestinal flora, eliminating toxic or inappropriate food groups from the daily diet, reducing stress and maintaining the sincere hope that the condition really can get better - all of these behaviours serve to encourage a more positive approach to the condition and instil a spirit of optimism that can make its own powerful contribution to the healing process.

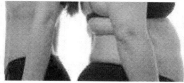

Chapter 3

ANTI INFLAMMATORY TACTICS and Epigenetics +
PALEO/KETO Eating Behaviours

The Anti-Inflammatory Diet is not a diet in the popular sense - it is not intended as a weight-loss program (although people can and do lose weight on it), nor is the Anti-Inflammatory Diet an eating plan to stay on for a limited period of time. Rather, it is way of selecting and preparing anti-inflammatory foods based on scientific knowledge of how they can help your body maintain optimum health. Along with influencing inflammation, this natural anti-inflammatory diet will provide steady energy and ample vitamins, minerals, essential fatty acids dietary fiber, and protective phytonutrients.

You can also adapt your existing recipes according to these anti-inflammatory diet principles:

General Diet tips

- Aim for variety.
- Include as much fresh food as possible.
- Minimize your consumption of processed foods and fast food.
- Eat an abundance of low sugar fruits and vegetables.

Caloric Intake

- Most adults need to consume between 2,000 and 3,000 calories a day.
- Women and smaller and less active people need fewer calories.
- Men and bigger and more active people need more calories.
- If you are eating the appropriate number of calories for your level of activity, your weight should not fluctuate greatly.
- The distribution of calories you take in should be as follows: 40 to 50 percent from carbohydrates, 30 percent from fat, and 20 to 30 percent from protein.
- Try to include carbohydrates, fat, and protein at each meal.

Carbohydrates

- On a 2,000-calorie-a-day diet, adult women should consume between 160 to 200 grams of carbohydrates a day.
- Adult men should consume between 240 to 300 grams of carbohydrates a day.
- The majority of this should be in the form of less-refined, less-processed foods with a low glycemic load.
- Stop ALL consumption of foods made with wheat flour and sugar, especially bread and most packaged snack foods (including chips and pretzels).
- Eat more winter squashes, and sweet potatoes.
- Cook only rice pasta al dente and eat it in moderation.
- Avoid products made with high fructose corn syrup.

Fat

- On a 2,000-calorie-a-day diet, 600 calories can come from fat - that is, about 67 grams. This should be in a ratio of 1:2:1 of saturated to monounsaturated to polyunsaturated fat.
- Reduce your intake of saturated fat by eating less butter, cream, high-fat cheese, unskinned chicken and fatty meats, and products made with palm kernel oil.
- Use extra-virgin olive oil as a main cooking oil. Organic, high-oleic, expeller pressed versions of sunflower and safflower oil are also acceptable.
- Avoid regular safflower and sunflower oils, corn oil, cottonseed oil, and mixed vegetable oils.
- Strictly avoid margarine, vegetable shortening, and all products listing them as ingredients. Strictly avoid all products made with partially hydrogenated oils of any kind. Include in your diet avocados and nuts, especially walnuts, cashews, almonds, and nut butters made from these nuts.
- For omega-3 fatty acids, eat salmon (preferably fresh or frozen wild or canned sockeye), sardines packed in water or olive oil, herring, and black cod (sablefish, butterfish); omega-3 fortified eggs; hemp seeds and flaxseeds (preferably freshly ground); or take a fish oil supplement (look for products that provide both EPA and DHA, in a convenient daily dosage of two to three grams).

Protein

- On a 2,000-calorie-a-day diet, your daily intake of protein should be between 80 and 120 grams. Eat less protein if you have liver or kidney problems, **allergies**, or autoimmune disease.
- Decrease your consumption of animal protein except for fish and high quality natural cheese and yogurt.
- Eat more vegetable protein, especially from hemp in particular. Become familiar with the range of veggie protein based foods available and find ones you like.

Fiber

- Try to eat 40 grams of fiber a day. You can achieve this by increasing your consumption of fruit, especially berries, vegetables (especially beans), and whole grains.
- Ready-made cereals can be good fiber sources, but read labels to make sure they give you at least 4 and preferably 5 grams of bran per one-ounce serving.

Phytonutrients

- To get maximum natural protection against age-related diseases (including cardiovascular disease, cancer, and neurodegenerative disease) as well as against environmental toxicity, eat a variety of fruits, vegetables and mushrooms.
- Choose fruits and vegetables from all parts of the color spectrum, especially berries, tomatoes, orange and yellow fruits, and dark leafy greens.
- Choose organic produce whenever possible. Learn which conventionally grown crops are most likely to carry pesticide residues and avoid them.
- Eat cruciferous (cabbage-family) vegetables regularly.
- Drink tea instead of coffee, especially good quality white, green or oolong tea.
- If you drink alcohol, use red wine preferentially.
- Enjoy plain dark chocolate in moderation (with a minimum cocoa content of 70 percent).

Vitamins and Minerals

The best way to obtain all of your daily vitamins, minerals, and micronutrients is by eating a diet high in fresh foods with an abundance of fruits and vegetables. In addition, supplement your diet with the following **antioxidant** cocktail:

- Vitamin C, 200 milligrams a day.
- Vitamin E, 400 IU of natural mixed tocopherols (d-alpha-tocopherol with other tocopherols, or, better, a minimum of 80 milligrams of natural mixed tocopherols and tocotrienols).
- Selenium, 200 micrograms of an organic (yeast-bound) form.
- Mixed carotenoids, 10,000-15,000 IU daily.
- The antioxidants can be most conveniently taken as part of a daily multivitamin/multimineral supplement that also provides at least 400 micrograms of folic acid and 2,000 IU of vitamin D. It should contain no iron (unless you are a female and having regular menstrual periods) and no preformed vitamin A (retinol). Take these supplements with your largest meal.
- Women should take supplemental calcium, preferably as calcium citrate, 500-700 milligrams a day, depending on their dietary intake of this mineral. Men should avoid supplemental calcium.

Other Dietary Supplements

- If you are not eating oily fish at least twice a week, take supplemental fish oil, in capsule or liquid form (two to three grams a day of a product containing both EPA and DHA). Look for molecularly distilled products certified to be free of heavy metals and other contaminants.
- Talk to your doctor about going on low-dose aspirin therapy, one or two baby aspirins a day (81 or 162 milligrams).
- If you are not regularly eating ginger and **turmeric**, consider taking these in supplemental form.
- Add **coenzyme Q10** (CoQ10) to your daily regimen: 60-100 milligrams of a softgel form taken with your largest meal.
- If you are prone to **metabolic syndrome**, take alpha-lipoic acid, 100 to 400 milligrams a day.

Water

- Drink pure water, or drinks that are mostly water (tea, very diluted fruit juice, sparkling water with lemon) throughout the day.
- Use bottled water or get a home water purifier if your tap water tastes of chlorine or other contaminants, or if you live in an area where the water is known or suspected to be contaminated.

One of the most common questions people with any form of arthritis have is, "Is there an arthritis diet?" Or more to the point, "What can I eat to help my joints?"

The answer, fortunately, is that many foods can help. Following a diet low in processed foods and saturated fat and rich in fruits, vegetables, fish, nuts and beans is great for your body. If this advice looks familiar, it's because these are the principles of the so-called Mediterranean diet, which is frequently touted for its anti-aging, disease-fighting powers.

Studies confirm eating these foods can do the following:

- Lower blood pressure

- Protect against chronic conditions ranging from cancer to stroke

- Help arthritis by curbing inflammation

- Benefit your joints as well as your heart

- Lead to weight loss, which makes a huge difference in managing joint pain.

Whether you call it a Mediterranean diet, an anti-inflammatory diet or simply an arthritis diet, here's a look at key foods to focus on – and why they're so good for joint health.

FIGHTING FIBROMYALGIA With THE ANTI- INFLAMMATORY DIET By Mercedes Del Rey

Fish

How much: Health authorities like The American Heart Association and the Academy of Nutrition and Dietetics recommend three to four ounces of fish, twice a week. Arthritis experts claim more is better.

Why: Some types of fish are good sources of inflammation-fighting omega-3 fatty acids. A study of 727 postmenopausal women, published in the *Journal of Nutrition* in 2004, found those who had the highest consumption of omega-3s had lower levels of two inflammatory proteins: C-reactive protein (CRP) and interleukin-6.

More recently, researchers have shown that taking fish oil supplements helps reduce joint swelling and pain, duration of morning stiffness and disease activity among people who have rheumatoid arthritis (RA).

Best sources: Salmon, tuna, sardines, herring, anchovies, scallops and other cold-water fish. Hate fish? Take a supplement. Studies show that taking 600 to 1,000 mg of fish oil daily eases joint stiffness, tenderness, pain and swelling.

Nuts & Seeds

How much: Eat 1.5 ounces of nuts daily (one ounce is about one handful).

Why: "Multiple studies confirm the role of nuts in an anti-inflammatory diet," explains José M. Ordovás, PhD, director of nutrition and genomics at the Jean Mayer USDA Human Nutrition Research Center on Aging at Tufts University in Boston.

A study published in *The American Journal of Clinical Nutrition* in 2011 found that over a 15-year period, men and women who consumed the most nuts had a 51 percent lower risk of dying from an inflammatory disease (like RA) compared with those who ate the fewest nuts. Another study, published in the journal *Circulation* in 2001 found that subjects with lower levels of vitamin B6 – found in most nuts – had higher levels of inflammatory markers.

More good news: Nuts are jam-packed with inflammation-fighting monounsaturated fat. And though they're relatively high in fat and calories, studies show noshing on nuts promotes weight loss because their protein, fiber and monounsaturated fats are satiating. "Just keep in mind that more is not always better," says Ordovás.

Best sources: Walnuts, pine nuts, pistachios and almonds.

Fruits & Veggies

How much: Aim for nine or more servings daily (one serving = 1 cup of most veggies or low sugar fruit or 2 cups raw leafy greens).

Why: Fruits and vegetables are loaded with antioxidants. These potent chemicals act as the body's natural defense system, helping to neutralize unstable molecules called free radicals that can damage cells.

FIGHTING FIBROMYALGIA With THE ANTI- INFLAMMATORY DIET By Mercedes Del Rey

Research has shown that anthocyanins found in cherries and other red and purple fruits like strawberries, raspberries, blueberries and blackberries have an anti-inflammatory effect.

Citrus fruits – like oranges, grapefruits and limes – are rich in vitamin C. Research shows getting the right amount of that vitamin aids in preventing inflammatory arthritis and maintaining healthy joints.

Other research suggests eating vitamin K-rich veggies like broccoli, spinach, lettuce, kale and cabbage dramatically reduces inflammatory markers in the blood.

Best sources: Colourful fruits and veggies – the darker or more brilliant the color, the more antioxidants it has. Good ones include blueberries, cherries, spinach, kale and broccoli.

Olive Oil

How much: Two to three tablespoons daily

Why: Olive oil is loaded with heart-healthy fats, as well as oleocanthal, which has properties similar to nonsteroidal, anti-inflammatory drugs. "This compound inhibits activity of COX enzymes, with a pharmacological action similar to ibuprofen," says Ordovás. Inhibiting these enzymes dampens the body's inflammatory processes and reduces pain sensitivity.

Best sources: Extra virgin olive oil goes through less refining and processing, so it retains more nutrients than standard varieties. And it's not the only oil with health benefits. Avocado and safflower oils have shown cholesterol-lowering properties while walnut oil has 10 times the omega-3s that olive oil has.

Grains

Should You Avoid Nightshades?

Nightshade vegetables, including eggplant, tomatoes, red bell peppers and potatoes, are disease-fighting powerhouses that boast maximum nutrition for minimal calories.

They also contain solanine, a chemical that has been branded the culprit in arthritis pain. There's no scientific evidence to suggest that nightshades trigger arthritis flares. In fact, some experts believe these vegetables contain a potent nutrient mix that helps inhibit arthritis pain.

However, many people do report significant symptom relief when they avoid nightshade vegetables. So doctors say, if you notice that your arthritis pain flares after eating them, do a test and try eliminating all nightshade vegetables from your diet for a few weeks to see if it makes a difference.

Epi – WHAT??

Perhaps you haven't heard all the excitement in medical and scientific circles about the latest revelations in the field of Epigenetics. Epi-what? OK. Before we go any further, you're probably wondering what on earth Epigenetics really means. Is it contagious? Can we get it at the grocery store?

FIGHTING FIBROMYALGIA With THE ANTI- INFLAMMATORY DIET By Mercedes Del Rey

Does it come in my size? So let's start by answering an important question: "What exactly is Epigenetics?"

The formal description of Epigenetics from the text books refers to the study of changes in organisms caused by modification of gene expression rather than by an alteration of the genetic code itself. That might not tell us very much but it really is an important statement! It's no longer simply a case of identifying which particular genes you have.

We now know that it's the way your genes are influenced and made to work that makes the difference. Gene expression accounts for so many of our characteristics. And changes in gene expression have been related to a very wide range of environmental influences and that includes – are you ready for this? – What we eat!

Yes, that's absolutely right. The kind of food we consume every single day, the quality of the food we eat, the eating choices we make all contribute far more to our total health and wellbeing than was ever appreciated before. It's not a question of being pre-programmed by our DNA. We've been bombarded by articles and news items for decades telling us every day that everything in our lives is caused by our genes.

But what if it isn't just the genetic luck of the draw? What if our health is connected far more to how we live, to what we eat and a whole range of external factors that we can influence? What if we're not programmed to be fat? What if it's about the choices we make? It's becoming increasingly clear that the choices we make really are incredibly important to our health and wellbeing. This means we really can influence our health right now right down to the cellular level and that obviously includes our weight as well. This is the breakthrough in our understanding that is revolutionising our entire approach to health and weight control. Our genes do not determine our weight. The answer is not in your genetic code. It's on the end of your fork!

So when we consult the latest reference works in this exciting new area of scientific research, we find that Epigenetics demonstrates the importance of influences which are firmly outside the traditional genetic system. This is the conclusion of Lyle Armstrong, whose research programme is widely respected at the Institute of Genetic Medicine at Newcastle University in the United Kingdom.

Modern biology is rewriting our understanding of genetics, disease and inherited characteristics. This is the view of Nessa Carey in her fascinating book "The Epigenetics Revolution".

This means that our understanding is also undergoing a revolution. The popular media still love to produce stories every day telling us that so many health problems are simply the result of your unlucky genes. But that's practically medieval in terms of medical science. We now know that we really can take the necessary steps to regain control of our general health, our health concerns and our weight. This must be one of the most important medical discoveries of the age.

Let's also bear in mind that science is not a fixed commodity.

In an age of extraordinary technological advances, our knowledge and understanding of how the human body functions are being tested and challenged every single day. That's why research is so important. And research changes the way we understand everything. This revolutionary development in our understanding of how the body really works is laying the foundation for all future medical analysis and treatment. The epigenetics principle represents one of the most important changes in how we are going to manage health issues in the future, from disease prevention to maintaining long term health.

The exciting thing is that we don't have to wait for the future to take full advantage of these discoveries. We are going to use it to get healthier and skinnier right now! We are going to show you the smart way to take control of your weight, and it's the way your body will love the most. We're going to help you to get into the best shape of your life. And we're going to show you how to stay that way.

Epigenetics Explained

The human body is made up of roughly 37 trillion cells, our structural building blocks. The "brain" of the cell is called the nucleus, and the nucleus contains our DNA. For years, we've assumed that DNA was a product of our heritage, handed down from mother and father, a rigid pre-determinant of everything from our height to our mathematical skills.

However, the revolutionary new field of *epigenetics* has led to the discovery that what we do actually changes the way our DNA is used, that the choices we make can forever *transform our genetic code*

This means that the way we interact with the world changes our DNA, not just the other way around. More intriguing, one of the major ways we can change our DNA is by diet. For example, a study published in 2008 showed that exposing mice brains to as little as 6 hours of high blood sugar led to epigenetic changes that increased risk of vascular damage.

These changes lasted even after 6 days of normal blood glucose, representing long-term damage after just a short blast of sugar. The research on long-term effects from short exposures is at the core of epigenetics. It's furthered by data from another 2008 study published in the journal *Diabetes*.

In this work, researchers showed that short periods of high blood glucose led to worse long term vascular changes than did sustained high blood glucose (a scary thought for the carbohydrate binger). Again, the underlying mechanism seems to be modification of the cell's DNA, leading to the extended duration of this effect.

But there's more. The most frightening data on this subject shows that high blood glucose may damage our telomeres; the ends of our DNA code. Considering that an undamaged telomere may be protective against cancer, death, and the very act of aging, any process that harms telomeres could put us at substantial risk. Data from the *Journal of Nutrition, Health and Aging* found that the higher the blood sugar, the more damage caused to the telomere and its associated DNA.

If we know that high levels of circulating glucose are trashing our DNA, it would make sense that diets low in glucose could have the opposite effect. Indeed, this is true. From the journal *Science*, the article "When Metabolism and Epigenetics Converge" relates the known neuroprotective benefits of a low carbohydrate diet to the epigenetic suppression of toxic oxidative stress.

This benefit, which was also seen with calorie restrictive diets, seems to indicate that choosing meals lower in carbohydrates and lower in calories improves our brain cells' ability to fight off damage, leading to healthier brains.

Epigenetics provides us with the insights, analysis, tools and strategies for permanent healthy weight loss.

Perhaps you've never heard about the excitement in medical and scientific circles about the latest revelations in the field of Epigenetics. But before we go any further, you're probably wondering what on earth Epigenetics really means. Is it contagious? Can we get it at the grocery store? Does it come in my size? So let's start by answering an important question: "What exactly is Epigenetics?"

The formal description of Epigenetics refers to the study of changes in organisms caused by modification of gene expression rather than by an alteration of the genetic code itself. That might not tell us very much but it really is an important statement! It's no longer simply a case of identifying which particular genes you have. We now know that it's the way your genes are influenced and made to work that makes the difference.

To start, we know that our genes definitely gave us a set of fixed characteristics. Eye colour, height and bone structure are examples of pre-determined characteristic donated by the genes you inherited from your parents.

But many areas of your life and wellbeing can be determined by the choices you make.

Weight control is a perfect example of this discovery. We now know that life span and the risk of contracting many diseases can be influenced by how we live our lives. The way we eat, the chemicals we absorb, the stress levels we endure all contribute to our health profiles and, most importantly, can change the way our DNA behaves. These minor alterations in gene behaviour can work in our favour or they can most certainly work against us. They can even be passed onto future generations.

So we have a direct responsibility for our own health and wellbeing and also for the welfare of future children and grandchildren. If you're interested in the technical background to this amazing phenomenon, the critical factor is a chemical code known as the epigenome.

This chemical coating surrounds your DNA and can switch certain genes off and on. So Epigenetics is primarily concerned with the study of this chemical layer and how it influences the way our genes function. Studies demonstrate that our genes only suggest what might happen in terms of our future health issues; our behaviour is much more important in determining the outcomes.

"There's nothing you can do about your DNA, but you can influence the way it functions by changing your lifestyle," says Ajay Goel, Ph.D., Director of Epigenetics and Cancer Prevention at Baylor Research Institute.

As a great example of how important this discovery has been for future health issues, even if you have a family history of certain kinds of cancer, eating particular foods can instruct the epigenome to switch off the cancer-prone genes.

You might want to read that sentence again.

The message is just too important to miss. This is the moment when the tide of obesity turns. This is when we recognise that we need to change our metabolic function as well as our food intake. This is when we finally take control of our weight issues. Now is the time to accept responsibility for our health and wellbeing and take the necessary steps to put things right. And keep them right.

If you're still keeping track of the technical data behind these revolutionary studies, you might like to know a little more about another influence on gene behaviour - methylation. This is a really interesting area of research but you might not want to make it your specialist subject when you go to parties! It's an incredibly important topic but most people, especially the ones who prefer to believe that they're just the unfortunate victims of their ill-fated DNA, probably don't want to have their illusions shattered. But you will know. And knowledge, my friend, especially this kind of knowledge is power.

Diet is a much easier subject to study than stress or other behaviours. It's been much easier to explore the effects of diet on epigenetics than the effects of the wider environment. So we know a great deal about the way food impacts on our genes.

Intelligent nutrition and appropriate exercise promote efficient fat-burning, healthy muscle building, longevity and wellness. Using your body's natural ability to respond to good nutrition, we can turn away forever from the nightmare of gaining and storing fat and losing muscle mass. We can reduce the risk of disease and illness. A brighter future beckons. This is the promise of Epigenetics.

As we mentioned before, our physical characteristics are largely based on our parents' DNA. Protecting your DNA from malfunction is not a luxury option any more. It's an essential task for all of us to undertake to ensure better health, quality of life and sustainable wellbeing.

Dr Trygve Tollefsbol wrote in the 2010 edition of Clinical Epigenetics that adding methyl-modifying compounds to the diet can help reduce the incidence and severity of disease. So we know from all the evidence that is being produced on a daily basis that you can reprogram your genes to favour weight loss, improve overall health and boost longevity by following three very simple procedures. You might want to print out these ideas and put them on your fridge door right now!

The PALEO-KETO <u>ANTI INFLAMMATORY</u> KETOGENIC EPIGENETIC EATING PROGRAM – what is it?

The PALEO-KETO Epigenetic Eating Three Golden Food Rules!

1. Weight loss is all about insulin

Moderate your insulin production levels by eliminating sugar and grains (yes, even whole grains) and you will lose the excess body fat without dieting - plus you will improve your energy levels, reduce inflammation throughout the body and eliminate disease risk. Maybe this should be printed in a very large font size in the brightest colour your printer can produce!

2. Eating lean…… protein but plenty good quality fat

Vegetable and some correctly sourced animal protein with high good fat content is not only healthy but is the key to effortless weight loss, a healthy immune system and boundless energy.

3. Eat Clean

When we examine the role that food plays in avoiding or encouraging weight gain, you might be shocked to discover that one of the biggest influences is concealed in the way that our food is processed. Hold onto your hat, my friend. This can get scary! The most significant components of food that play the largest role in weight gain and obesity are food additives, chemicals, and food processing techniques.

These principles are sacred and mark the beginning of your transformation. They are so important that they need to be practised and respected every single day. They are the foundation for much of the change we are creating. You could finish the book first but the only time you have to begin the revolution is right now. So let's make the commitment right this instant to use these golden principles and kick start the new life we've been waiting for. And I mean right now!

Epigenetic research has been at the forefront of these discoveries and that's why the methods in this book respect the need to resolve all of the issues surrounding intelligent, effective, permanent weight control.

So many people find that even when they've managed to lose some weight, it goes back on in a flash. We did not evolve to be chronically overweight. Nature equipped us with incredibly efficient bodies. Clearly we need a better approach to this problem. We need an approach that works. We need a method that will give us sustainable results. So let's take a look at some of the more recent innovations in weight control technology.

It's time to get some much needed clarity into the discussion. So, let's begin by asking – What exactly is the Ketogenic Diet?

FIGHTING FIBROMYALGIA With THE ANTI- INFLAMMATORY DIET By Mercedes Del Rey
KETOGENICS

We're going to start by defining precisely what ketosis is and why it's so important for so many aspects of our health and wellbeing, and that includes sustainable weight loss too.

Ketosis (pronounced KEY-TOE-SIS) is a word that describes the metabolic state that occurs when you consume a very low-carb, moderate-protein, high-fat diet. Ketosis causes your body to switch from using glucose as its primary source of fuel to running on ketones. Ketones themselves are produced when the body burns fat, and they're primarily used as an alternative fuel source when glucose isn't available.

In other words, in the simplest and most dramatic way of summing up the process, your body changes from a sugar-burner to a fat-burner. Depending on your current diet and lifestyle choices, getting into ketosis can take as little as a few days and or as much as several weeks. In some cases it's even taken months. So "being in ketosis" just means that you are burning fat. You might need some good, old-fashioned, patience and persistence but the range of benefits absolutely justifies the effort as you pursue ketosis.

If you have ever fasted by skipping breakfast after a good night's sleep, then you likely have begun producing trace amounts of ketones in your blood. The secret to the process is remarkably simple in its concept: you consume a diet with very few carbohydrates, moderate levels of protein, and plenty of healthy, saturated and monounsaturated fats. This combination encourages an increase in the number of ketones produced in your body, until they dominate the way your body is fuelled, even to the point that you need very little glucose to function with lots of energy available to you.

Dr. William Wilson, a family practitioner and expert on nutrition and brain function, explained that "throughout most of our evolutionary history, humans used both glucose and ketone bodies for energy production." He said that our Paleolithic ancestors used glucose as their body's preferred fuel when non-animal food was available. But during periods of food shortages or when animal-based foods were their primary source of calories, our ancestors spent most of their time in a state of ketosis. He added, "If our early ancestors hadn't developed a way to use ketones for energy, our species would have ended up on Darwin's short list eons ago!"

Ketone bodies provide an alternative fuel for the brain, heart, and most other organs when serum glucose and insulin levels are low—i.e., on a very low-carbohydrate diet. Ketone bodies are actually preferred over glucose by the heart and can be used as efficiently as glucose by most portions of the brain. There is a growing body of research supporting their beneficial effects on ageing, inflammation, metabolism, cognition, and athletic performance.

Once you begin to consider the advantages of having higher levels of ketones in your body, you soon realise that they are the preferred fuel source for the muscles, heart, liver, and brain. These vital organs do not handle carbohydrates very well; in fact, they become damaged when we consume too many carbs.

According to Dr. Ron Rosedale, ketones themselves are a great, and in many tissues—such as the brain—far better, fuel source than the conventional, glucose alternative.

Ketosis is also an excellent way to lose body fat. Ketones are merely a by-product of burning fat for fuel. In other words, burning fat generates ketones at the same time. When you are keto-adapted, you generate energy from both your body fat and dietary fat. However, when you consume excess carbohydrates, they are converted into body fat, which cannot be easily accessed to provide fuel for the body. This is another great reason for you to be in a ketogenic state. It's one of the human body's most effective mechanisms for burning excess fat.

Let's just repeat that message one more time. A low-carb, high-fat, ketogenic diet is a very powerful and highly effective fat-burning process that's especially useful for anyone who is overweight or obese. Weight issues tend to respond extremely well to a ketogenic approach, too. After all, it's hard to become efficient at burning body fat if you're busy burning sugar and starch all the time. Now you can see why all those carbs have been at the heart of so many weight issues.

Here are some of the many health benefits that come from being in ketosis: (DISCLAIMER – Some of these benefits may be hampered by poor health and lifestyle choices in other areas than diet!)

- Natural hunger and appetite control
- Effortless weight loss and maintenance
- Mental clarity
- Sounder, more restful sleep
- Normalized metabolic function
- Stabilized blood sugar and restored insulin sensitivity
- Lower inflammation levels
- Feelings of happiness and general well-being
- Lowered blood pressure
- Increased HDL (good) cholesterol
- Reduced triglycerides
- Lowered or eliminated small LDL particles (bad cholesterol)
- Use of stored body fat as a fuel source
- Improved immune system
- Slowed aging due to reduction in free radical production
- Improvements in blood chemistry
- Optimized cognitive function and improved memory
- Heightened understanding of how foods affect your body
- Faster and better recovery from exercise
- Decreased anxiety and mood swings

So if ketosis is so desirable, then haven't the health authorities been at the forefront of the campaign to help people experience the enormous benefits of the system? It's a valid question because the subject has been labelled with an undeserved negative reputation, which is especially unfortunate considering all the countless lives that it could improve. As with many things in life, it comes down to fear and a chronic lack of knowledge and education amongst the medical professionals. It stems primarily from a simple misunderstanding of what ketosis really means.

Part of the problem lies in the word ketosis itself, which closely resembles ketoacidosis, a medical term that's used to describe a life-threatening condition in type 1 diabetics. Many doctors scoff at the idea of allowing one of their patients to get into a state of ketosis because they immediately think of all the negative side effects associated with ketoacidosis. This confusion may have allowed many patients to remain in a diseased state when they could have seen tremendous improvements in their health with the use of a ketogenic diet. It's a sad reality that this kind of ignorance happens in the medical profession, with the very people we trust to be our purveyors of knowledge on health.

Jackie Eberstein says (see references)

"Nutritional ketosis is not ketoacidosis. Yet many in the medical profession have a knee-jerk reaction to ketones. Their knowledge is limited and possibly biased. "

Here's why doctors are so concerned about ketoacidosis: When diabetics do not get an adequate amount of insulin, their bodies respond as if they are starving. Their bodies think there's no more glucose to be had, either from diet or glycogen stores, and they switch to burning fat instead and ramp up ketone production so it can be used as an alternative energy source. The problem is, these diabetics aren't out of glucose—in fact, they have elevated levels of blood glucose. Insulin is the hormone that allows glucose into cells, and without it, the blood sugar has nowhere to go and accumulates in the bloodstream, even as the body can't stop making ketones. It's an extremely serious thing and certainly should not be messed around with. But keep in mind this condition only applies to type 1 diabetics and, very rarely, truly insulin-dependent type 2 diabetics.

It would be impossible for this sequence of events to happen to non-diabetics. If you can produce even a small amount of insulin in your body, ketones naturally remain at safe levels.

You may have heard that ketosis is a "dangerous state" for the body to be in. But ketosis simply means that your body is metabolizing a high amount of natural, fat-based energy sources. Ketones are molecules generated during fat metabolism—and that can be fat from the avocado you just ate or fat from the adipose tissue around your middle.

HOWEVER – NEVER START THIS DIET WITHOUT PRIOR PERMISSION OF A CERTIFIED MEDICAL PROFESSIONAL WELL VERSED IN THE UNDERSTANDING OF THE BENEFITS OF KETOSIS!

Doctors Are Using Ketogenic Diets with Great Success

Dr Terry Wahls states: (see references)

FIGHTING FIBROMYALGIA With THE ANTI- INFLAMMATORY DIET By Mercedes Del Rey

"Humans went into ketosis every winter for thousands of generations. Being in a low level of ketosis is the more natural state for our metabolism. We do have metabolic flexibility and can operate on amino acids, glucose or fat."

Many doctors are prescribing a low-carb, high-fat nutritional approach for patients who are dealing with a wide variety of chronic health problems, and they are seeing dramatic improvements in patient health based on the new approach to diet.

For example....It wasn't until Dr. Sue Wolver hit middle age herself that she realized why her patients were so unsuccessful on her prescribed low-fat diet. She suddenly found, she said, that "my own advice didn't even work for me!" (see references)

"Despite my adherence to a low-fat diet and exercise, every time I got on the scale I weighed more," Dr. Wolver explained. "That's when I first started thinking the advice I had been giving might actually be wrong."

Dr. Wolver's breakthrough moment of understanding occurred when she heard physician and researcher Dr. William S. Yancy, Jr., give a talk entitled "Taking the Fat Out of the Fire," in which he discussed the health benefits of a low-carb, high-fat, ketogenic approach to nutrition. She "was hooked." Dr. Wolver immediately began putting herself into a state of ketosis and the weight poured off and stayed off, and all without the intense hunger she had previously experienced. These days, she uses herself as a prime example for her patients of how ketogenic diets can help them with their weight and health issues.

Nora Gedgaudus says ...."I have seen mood stabilization, reduced or eliminated depression, reduced or eliminated anxiety, improved cognitive functioning, greatly enhanced and evened-out energy levels, cessation of seizures, improved overall neurological stability, cessation of migraines, improved sleep, improvement in autistic symptoms, improvements with PCOS (polycystic ovary syndrome), improved gastrointestinal functioning, healthy weight loss, cancer remissions and tumor shrinkage, much better management of underlying previous health issues, improved symptoms and quality of life in those struggling with various forms of autoimmunity (including many with type 1 and 1.5 diabetes), fewer colds and fius, total reversal of chronic fatigue, improved memory, sharpened cognitive functioning, and significantly stabilized temperament. And there is quality evidence to support the beneficial impact of a fat-based ketogenic approach in all these types of issues. "

- Nora Gedgaudas (see references)

It is Essential to Find Your Carbohydrate Tolerance Level

Maria Emmerich says ""Everyone is different and has different carb-tolerance levels. Some people, especially athletes, can maintain ketosis with as much as 100 grams of carbs a day. But most people need to be at 50 grams or less, and those with metabolic syndrome typically need to stay below 30 grams of total carbs a day to produce adequate ketones.

- Maria Emmerich (see references)

Franziska Spritzler says "At lower carbohydrate and protein intakes, the percentage of calories coming from fat increases even if the amount does not change. Most people in nutritional ketosis consume anywhere from 65 to 80 percent of their calories as fat. "

-

At this point it would be impossible for anyone to give you a specific amount of carbohydrates to consume in order to get into ketosis. You can only determine that figure through personal experimentation under close medical supervision. But once you figure out your carb tolerance, you'll be well on your way to paleo – keto - epigenetic success.

Adapted from: Moore, Jimmy, and Dr. Eric Westman, Keto Clarity

---

The Paleo Diet

The theory is that many of our current health problems are a result of our modern eating habits. There's been a great deal of publicity surrounding the growing view that we simply haven't evolved to the point where we can safely consume a grain-rich diet. Our distant ancestors in the Old Stone Age or Paleolithic Era consumed a very different diet compared to modern humans because they simply didn't have access to agriculture. That's because agriculture didn't exist. It hadn't been invented. The typical caveman's food was natural, unprocessed, varied, seasonal and a result of labour-intensive, hunter-gathering activities.

The Paleo approach to nutrition recognises that we've only been consuming grains for the last ten thousand years or so. That's a long wait at the bus stop but it really is not long enough in evolutionary terms for humans to have adapted to this radical shift in eating behaviour. The modern diet is heavily reliant on grains and dairy products and suffers from a toxic surfeit of sugar. Grains were the mechanism that allowed for a more predictable food supply and those ancient crop surpluses provided the essential catalyst from which the seeds of civilisation sprang. The problem, as you now know only too well, is that grains damage the gut, weaken the immune system and degrade our health.

The Paleo alternative recognises how our digestive system works and focuses on providing the best quality fuel for our bodies. That includes fresh fruits, vegetables, lean meat, eggs and nuts. No grains. No processed sugars. No milk products. Paleo has scored very highly as a weight control mechanism because this kind of diet suits our evolutionary history so well. When we adapt our eating habits to this more natural way of getting our daily calories, our metabolisms shift from carb-burning to fat-burning. No surprise then that the Paleo diet has become a favourite tool for encouraging serious weight loss and for enhancing better levels of health.

The focus is on natural, unprocessed food and it is this emphasis on eating as naturally as possible that is the key to the method's success. As you might expect in a new way of approaching our food needs, the Paleo diet has spawned a number of variations and alternatives. Some enthusiasts avoid all forms of dairy produce whilst others are convinced that some specific dairy products are essential. The wisdom of avoiding grains though is widely accepted by most Paleo devotees.

You might recognise some aspects of the Paleo Diet in our advice in this book. It certainly has some interesting and relevant merits in terms of getting the body into great shape and the emphasis on pure protein and natural, unprocessed vegetables is a key to restoring the intestinal flora to its healthiest and most effective condition.

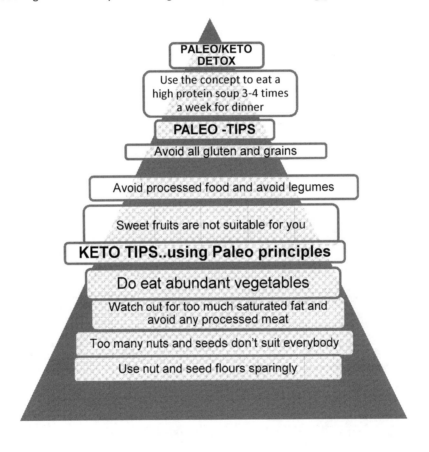

PALEO/KETO DETOX
Use the concept to eat a high protein soup 3-4 times a week for dinner

PALEO -TIPS
Avoid all gluten and grains

Avoid processed food and avoid legumes

Sweet fruits are not suitable for you

KETO TIPS..using Paleo principles

Do eat abundant vegetables

Watch out for too much saturated fat and avoid any processed meat

Too many nuts and seeds don't suit everybody

Use nut and seed flours sparingly

Summary - Epigenetics

Your genetic profile is not the full story

Your genes can be switched on and off

The food you eat is the key to influencing your genetic responses

Methylation and diet change the rules of the genetic game

Managing insulin levels by eliminating all grains

Eat Lean, Clean and Good fats

Take practical steps to address food addiction

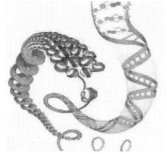

Chapter 4

The Epigenetic Mythbuster Chart

The Epigenetic Mythbuster Chart.....your 5 point blueprint and lifelong passport to the happy realm of total weight control and permanent residence in the Land of Leaner.

CMR Conventional Medical Recommendation.

DEFINITION: The old view of what is supposed to be good for you.

EPS Epigenetic Paradigm Shift.

DEFINITION: The revolutionary new advances in medical and scientific research that will transform your health

Let's get serious. Fact: If the old ways worked, we wouldn't be having an explosion of obesity in the developed world and we wouldn't be having this conversation, would we? Clearly something is missing. Our mission is to show you what the problem really is, how to fix the problem and fix it forever.

Step 1: Grains

> *CMR:* Insists that grains are actually good for you. Wheat, rice, corn, cereal, bread, pasta etc. Most governments recommend 8-10 servings per day as the principle daily source of energy, nutrition and fiber. Entire industries are devoted to promoting this idea as the healthiest way to live. Ask pretty much anyone and they'll tell you how good it is to eat grains.

> *EPS:* UCLA lecturer and world famous evolutionary biologist Jared Diamond stipulates "Grains are the worst mistake of the human race." In nutritional terms, grains are simply inferior to plants. Grains trigger insulin production and fat storage.

They produce allergic reactions, suppress the immune response and trigger a wide range of intolerances as well as imbalances in the intestinal flora.

Step 2: Fats

CMR: Fat makes you fat therefore if you reduce fat you'll lose fat. The world is awash with countless 'fat free' and 'low fat' products and we have a ballooning obesity problem.

EPS: Good quality fat drives efficient fat and protein metabolism, encouraging weight loss and boosting energy levels.

Step 3: Meal Habits

CMR: Three square meals a day plus snacks are best to stave off hunger pangs and stabilize metabolism

EPS: Any steps to normalize your insulin production encourages your skinny genes to take over. Occasional fasting using protein soup meals can help you to reprogram your fat burning potential

Step 4: Cardio exercise

CMR: 30-60 minutes cardio per day. Lift weights regularly using isolated parts of the body and aim for maximum resistance, even going for the point of failure to increase strength.

EPS: Weight resistance using the whole body in short bursts plus slower more regular cardio exercise for shorter periods per day with sporadic intense bursts of intensity. This system really does work!

Step 5: Sun exposure

CMR: Wear sunscreen every day, in all weather and in every season. It should have a sun protection factor (SPF) of 30 and say "broad-spectrum" on the label, which means it protects against the sun's UVA and UVB rays. Put it on at least 15 minutes before going outside. Use 1 ounce, which would fill a shot glass

EPS: Sunshine can be a tricky thing. We need it, but it can also be harmful.

Striking the right balance between getting enough sunshine to produce optimal levels of Vitamin D, and protecting ourselves from the harm the sun can do, can be a challenge. Most experts recommend 15-20 minutes of sun exposure several times a week for the average fair-skinned person, as this is enough to produce optimal levels of Vitamin D while not being so much to damage skin. Darker skin tones with more melanin need to stay in the sun longer to synthesize vitamin D effectively...see more info below

Vitamin D, which our body produces when we are exposed to sunlight, does wonders for us – from improving mood to boosting our immune systems, reducing inflammation and much more, it's key to our health.

According to some new research, it seems there is yet another reason to get the right amount of sunlight. Researchers found that older women (65+) with low Vitamin D levels are more likely to gain weight.

Time Bomb Triggers

It's very controversial but it looks increasingly likely that humans made a massive and deeply influential error around seven thousand years ago. It wasn't intended as an error. It happened because it looked exactly like a brilliant strategy for survival. In fact the idea was so good that it rapidly spread and became the foundation for human civilisation. The brilliant idea was agriculture.

Brilliant because it helped to solve the constant challenge of ensuring a regular food supply. A profound error because it encouraged our ancestors to become completely dependent on grains. Seven thousand years ago is effectively yesterday in evolutionary terms. Our bodies did not evolve to exist on a grain-rich diet. But that is what has happened over the last seven thousand years.

The human genome hasn't changed very much during this time span but our diet and lifestyle have diverged dramatically from the way our ancestors lived before the introduction of agriculture. It is believed that many of our contemporary diseases have arisen as a result of this revolution in our dietary habits.

We'll take a closer look at these important issues as we explore the great behaviours you can use to transform your weight and your life. For now let's concentrate on the more obvious consequences of the way we eat.

You've probably already guessed the most obvious outcome of these changes in our diet; an astonishing increase in disease at a time of unprecedented medical advances. Scientists are beginning to suspect a common cause to this tendency towards disease: it's all in our diet. Seven thousand years might not have been long enough for humans to have adapted successfully to a grain-oriented diet. And then, of course, we have the strange phenomenon of obesity. The problem, like many waistlines, is getting bigger.

In 1980 there were approximately 875 million overweight and obese people in the world. In 2013, the number had grown to 2.1 billion. That's an increase of 28% in adult obesity and, more alarmingly, a 47% increase in the number of overweight children in just the past thirty-three years. What could be causing such a radical shift in the average size and weight of humans in such a dramatically short period of time? The answer might lie within us. Or, to be more precise, within our gut.

45

FIGHTING FIBROMYALGIA With THE ANTI- INFLAMMATORY DIET By Mercedes Del Rey

Recent discoveries about the trillions of microorganisms that live in and on the human body are now changing the traditional perspective on human health and disease. In terms of obesity, we're learning that it's not just heredity and gene expression related to our human genome that play a role, but also the trillions of microorganisms that make up the vastly larger (in terms of unique genetic material) second genome in our body, the human microbiome. Studies have begun to describe each human gut as a highly complex eco-system, populated by communities of bacteria as well by viruses, fungi and moulds. The contents of our gut seem to exert an extraordinary influence on our digestive system, but these micro flora also affect our health in general, our wellbeing and even our mental and emotional balance. Imbalances in the micro flora of the gut have now been identified as an important cause of obesity. The gut's microbiome, that miniature universe within our digestive system, is where many of our health and weight issues are focused.

The obese gut microcosm

One of the disorders that we now know is associated with an altered gut microflora is obesity. There is a wealth of fascinating evidence from initial studies that reveal a distinct connection between the microbes in our gut and the way our bodies regulate fat storage. These results have been widely replicated and numerous other reports have confirmed this relationship. By now it's well established that obesity is characterised by an obese-oriented microbiota and that gut microbes really can influence fat storage through a variety of mechanisms.

Adding depth to our understanding of the obesity problem, we know that obesity is virtually unheard of in hunter-gatherer populations and the same observation holds true for many non-westernised societies. So we can conclude that obesity is predominantly a disease of civilised, grain-consuming societies. There's a major clue here about some of the causes of unhealthy weight gain that dominate developed societies.

We can look a little deeper into this question about the influence of our gut flora. Obese or overweight people have different gut flora compared to lean individuals. Yes they do. Hunter gatherers also have a very different microbiome compared to the intestinal flora of westernised peoples. And we know that hunter gatherers don't do fat! It also seems clear that flora in the gut can influence metabolic hormones such as leptin and insulin, key influencers in the body's inflammatory response. Research is identifying the extraordinary role of prebiotics, probiotics and other microbiome stabilisers in encouraging fat loss in humans and animals. Surprised? Utterly amazed that changing and re-balancing your gut flora can be so beneficial for your health and weight loss issues? Stay with me, my friend. We're just getting started!

More on the importance of correct sun exposure.

Vitamin D, which our body produces when we are exposed to sunlight, does wonders for us – from improving mood to boosting our immune systems, reducing inflammation and much more, it's key to our health. According to some new research, it seems there is yet another reason to get the right amount of sunlight. Researchers found that older women (65+) with low Vitamin D levels are more likely to gain weight

Folks, without question, the best way to get the right amount of vitamin D is to spend some time in the sun.

You always want to avoid getting burned, but generally speaking you can safely spend anywhere from 20 minutes to two hours in the sun every day with beneficial effects. If you have dark-colored skin or live far from the equator, you will need to spend more time in the sun than someone who is light-skinned living close to the equator.

There are many available books and studies on the benefits and risks of too sunlight and vitamin d depletion. Contact me for a recommend reading list at beranparry@gmail.com

It's becoming clear now that the pathway to sustainable health and wellbeing, to a leaner, fitter, stronger and happier body is not in the outdated Conventional Medical Recommendations. The future is in the Epigenetics Revolution and the Skinny Paradigm Shift.

Summary - Mythbuster

The folly of grains in the human diet

Welcome to the inner universe of your microbiome

Being overweight is closely connected to the state of your gut flora

CMR versus EPS (epigenetic paradigm shift)

EPS - The smarter way to live long, lose weight and live better

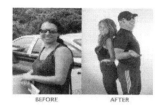

BEFORE   AFTER

Chapter5

Getting Organised to make Epigenetic Eating Behaviour more Effective!

5 Steps to Re Organising Your Permanent Weight Reduction and Leaner Pathway!

Time to re-programme your food choices and eating behaviour

We are going to learn how to:

Exorcise the past and be free of old habits

Why we prioritise our activities in the wrong order

I've heard it so often, it's almost become the mantra of the unwilling, the permanent excuse for letting things slide. "There just isn't enough time to eat healthily and plan special meals, let alone shop or cook them or take them with me when I'm out of the house."

Sound familiar? ...here are more excuses.....

I feel so awful when I've eaten badly.

I feel such a failure.

My life is a mess.

Why is it such a struggle to lose weight?"

The result is a fairly miserable outlook and a lack of confidence, an unwillingness to recognise what is possible. The mind-set of the victim. But we're here to address these issues. We want you to feel the confidence that comes from daily, planned success. And getting organised takes all the pain and doubt from the process.

The irony is that the people who claim there's no time to incorporate these important changes in their lives have often been completely successful in other areas of their lives. Their success shows up in an infinite number of ways: they were incredibly accomplished managers or employees, highly creative artistic individuals, massively good parents or even someone who was good at something else. Every time you make a decision to do something, you're engaging your creative power. All we have to do is harness that potential.

Unhappiness can undoubtedly play its part in the way we treat our bodies. If you have doubts about your self-worth - I know, welcome to the human condition! - It often shows up in unhealthy eating habits and poor choices. It's a huge area and so important that it will be the subject of a future book.

That's why I'd like to encourage you to do something incredibly powerful right now. I want you to look in the mirror for a few moments. And smile. That's right. Smile. Look at yourself and smile. Your conscious mind might feel that the act is a little silly but your subconscious - and your body - will begin to get the message that you're giving them your personal stamp of approval. Have you ever noticed how a small child lights up when you really smile at them? Your body needs exactly that same recognition, that same high wattage smile of approval. Do it every time you step into the bathroom. Look into the mirror and smile. The results will amaze you.

We want your body and your subconscious to work with you. Give them that dazzling smile and you will find your body begins to co-operate in the most extraordinary ways. Try it. It's a very powerful technique for removing behavioural obstacles and we want to make this entire process as easy and comfortable as possible.

This entire book is designed to help you take control of your health, your weight and ultimately your happiness. Being kind to yourself, respecting the miracle of your body, learning to enjoy living in such an extraordinary structure, optimising its potential and being at peace with yourself. These are powerful keys to a very fulfilling way of experiencing the gift of life.

So the underlying theme to these methods is to be kind to yourself. To do things that benefit rather than harm your health. To respect your body's needs and live life to the full.

An abiding love and acceptance of yourself, despite all the imperfections, really helps you to overcome any harmful habits and behaviours and puts an end to the self-criticism and self-loathing that lowers self esteem and sabotages our efforts. It really is extraordinary how quickly we can change our lives simply by learning to accept ourselves and focus not on what might be amiss but on how we truly want to be.

1. Identify your behaviours and habits.

Take a moment. Listen to that inner voice, the way you speak to yourself; check the way you feed yourself; think about your hygiene and sleeping habits.

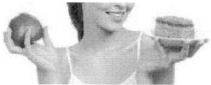

Which of these areas makes you feel uncomfortable in any way?

Here were a few examples

Allowing yourself to eat unhealthy food because there just wasn't the time or opportunity to make the effort

Believing that the needs of others are more important than taking care of your body and your weight

Eating food that isn't good for you at any time

Eating late at night or just eating too much

Eating while standing up, out of the package, staring at a computer screen or watching TV

If you catch yourself in the cycle of doing something that you really know you shouldn't, it's an important indicator that there are unresolved issues at work in the subconscious that continue to influence your behaviour.

2. Think about the real consequences of your behaviour.

You might discover that these behaviours and habits are very effective at preventing you from having the things you really want, particularly in terms of having a fit and healthy body that you can really appreciate.

In every moment we are thinking, feeling and doing things that either bring us closer to the person we want to be and the life we want to have or our behaviours take us away from those precious possibilities.

Behaviours ultimately reflect how we really feel about ourselves. Learn to accept yourself right now and the process of transformation will flow so much more smoothly. Learn to smile at yourself and your deeper resources will turn their power towards your new, healthier goals and desires.

3. Learn to understand where your habits came from.

So much of our behaviour was laid down during our early childhoods that we completely forget how we came to be the way we are. Much of our conditioning is no more than a series of programmed reflexes that were given to us at a very impressionable age and those behaviours have survived in our attitudes, thoughts, feelings and beliefs ever since.

Whether they are entirely appropriate can only be measured in terms of whether you're really experiencing all the health, self-expression and happiness that is available to you. Most people are not. Sad. But true. Take a look around you. Not too many happy smiling faces, are there? I rest my case. If you're feeling unhappy, comfort is something that is obviously missing and food is one of the easiest sources of a temporary quick fix.

Yes. We're talking chocolate here! So many people reach for the chocolate for an instant rush of pleasure, a way to escape the reality of a stressed and unfulfilled life. Pure comfort food. And I like chocolate too. The intention always seems positive. You give yourself a measure of much needed comfort and an ounce of joy. Unfortunately, it isn't the healthiest way to give yourself those things and it comes with the undesired effects of insulin spikes, sugar crashes and inevitable weight gain followed by a bout of guilt and quiet despair! There has to be a better way. (There is a better way to eat chocolate too...I promise!)

As adults, we're expected to understand the consequences of engaging in a particular thought or behaviour but we often do it anyway. The motivation is always moving away from pain or increasing pleasure. And so many of these actions are a product of that early (and now unconscious) conditioning. It's as if the adult has to be driven so often by a rebellious four year old! No wonder much of our behaviour doesn't make sense. No wonder we don't always behave like truly responsible grownups.

Comfort food can be very satisfying. We know that many unhealthy behaviours feel good in the short-term (the sugar rush, the comfort, the satisfaction) but we have to recognise that they have long-term detrimental effects. There can also be that familiar hint of the rebel, the thrill of ignoring good advice and breaking the rules. What is it about ourselves that prompts us to do really things to our bodies?

Awareness is very helpful in these circumstances. Spotting the moment when you get a kick from doing the wrong thing helps you to question what's really happening. The adult gets a chance to intervene and make a better choice. That moment when you pause for an instant and wonder why you're doing something, even wondering who is really making the decision. Consciously and deliberately making a wiser, healthier choice. Feeling really good because you've done the right thing. A positive feedback loop that reinforces good behaviour, good choices, adult decisions.

4. Create "house meal planning and eating rules."

Parents make rules because they understand that their children might not have the right perspective for good judgement. Parents can see the consequences that are usually beyond the child's range of experience.

If you have a particularly hard habit to break and you know it's not good for your well-being, consider making it a "house rule" never to have that habit in the home. When something is non-negotiable it removes the inner dialogue where we bargain with ourselves and the simple rule reinforces the right decisions...

5. Develop your powers of awareness.

Be kind to yourself. Most people don't respond well to punishment. Treat yourself gently and with consideration. You've embarked on an important journey and that requires courage and a large measure of recognition.

Be infinitely patient with yourself, as you would be with a child. If you slip up once, instead of throwing everything out the window, learn to accept the failure and resolve to do better.

Understand why you did what you did. What did you need in that moment? Use your new set of rules to support your new behaviour. The rules are your friends. They are there to help you.

What are your new "house eating rules"? How can you maintain your new habits in a way that is supportive, effective and nurturing?

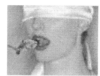

Here are some examples

1. I always make sure that I have the healthy foods I love at home by doing the shopping myself or by having someone do the shopping for me

2. I always make sure that I have a healthy snack available to me in my refrigerator at all times

3 I always call restaurants ahead of time to order my personal food requirements so that I won't feel uncomfortable when I get there

4. I always take healthy snacks with me to avoid temptation

5. I never allow myself to get too hungry and then I won't have an excuse to eat unhealthy food

These tried and tested methods allow you to exercise control over your feelings and your environment, removing many of the challenging decisions about food choices by making one powerful, healthy choice for all future situations. As you become more aware of how you feel, catching yourself thinking, feeling and about to do things that are no longer in line with your new commitment to total health, you can let go of the old behaviour and make really great choices that will support your vision of a newer, healthier, happier, skinnier you!

To give you some ideas about typical eating behaviour choices, we've prepared a list of situations to see if any of them partly or completely describe your own personal reactions. Remember, you're the only person who'll see the answers so be honest with yourself. It isn't a test. It's just a lens to help us focus more clearly on the issues.

Please tick those statements that apply to you – even a tiny bit!

1. When you eat out at restaurants that have buffets you often overeat. You find it hard to eat in moderation at these restaurants. You find yourself getting seconds and thirds in this situation.

2. You are feeling really hungry and start to panic that you really need to eat something...so you grab the first available snack because you are REALLY hungry....

3. This is a very busy time in your life. You are always rushed. You don't have time to cook the right types of food let alone plan them. It seems as if everything that you have time to cook is not allowed on your meal plan. You feel as if you are locked into a never ending cycle. When you don't eat right, you feel bad, and when you feel bad, you don't like to eat right.

4. During the week you have a very structured routine but sometimes on the weekends your routine is less structured making meal planning difficult. Often you eat the wrong types of food because you do not plan your meals.

5. You have evening activities that prevent you eating a healthy dinner. So you just grab whatever is available and convince yourself "it's just the once".

6. You are visiting friends for a meal or your vacation. These friends cook with butter and fat and have a cake or pie for dessert every night. You feel that you must eat what is served or not eat at all. You do not feel comfortable asking for foods that fit into your meal plan.

7. You are on your way to an important meeting and are running late. If you do not get stopped by any more lights, you will just make the meetings. You look down and see that bag of unhealthy snacks that you picked up this morning. Sometimes you get stressed out; eating something seems to make you feel better. You are tempted to eat the snacks

8. You have had an awful day. You were in line for a promotion or a new contract and your best friend or a competitor got it instead of you. When you went to pick up the laundry at the dry cleaners they had lost it. Then, you got a flat tire only three blocks from home. You feel like "pigging out". You don't care what you're supposed to eat. You are really depressed and you think that you deserve something special.

9. You are planning on going to the movies tonight with your friends. Your favourite treat is buttered popcorn and the movie theatre is running a special on large popcorn and free refills on large drinks. What would you do at a sports event in this situation?....just wade in and join the feeding frenzy?

Even if there was just one tick, there is room for improvement, because just that one item of behavioural change can make a huge difference to your permanent weight loss outcome!

NOW

Log on to our website and take the Epigenetic Eating Behaviour Test and see if your score is over 100 or less...or is it over 150 or even 200..check out your final score results at the end

www.skinnydeliciouslife.com/eating-behaviour-questionnaire

EATING BEHAVIOUR TIPS!

1. I stop for a fast food breakfast on the way to work.
There's no substitute for a good, healthy breakfast. Probably the most important meal of the day.

2. My emotions affect what and how much I eat
Learn to breathe more deeply. I'm serious. Slow down and deepen your breathing and you'll relax more, reducing the need to snack on sugary killer foods

3. I use low-fat food products
This is not the right choice because low fat normally means high sugar

4. I am not careful about the portion sizes of my foods.
Slow down and take your time when you're eating. Stop. Think about how much food you really need. Be aware of your choices.

5. I buy snacks from vending machines.
Arm yourself with healthy snacks at the start of the day so you won't be tempted to purchase poison from a vending machine.

6. I choose foods without a thought about heart disease.
Knowledge is power, my friend. This workbook has prepared you with the knowledge to spot those killer foods that attack your heart. Now you can successfully avoid them and become healthier.

7. I never eat meatless meals because I think that is healthier for me.
The old argument about processed food applies here too. It isn't meat per se that's the problem. It's the hormones, antibiotics and chemicals that are pumped into the animals to fatten them up for slaughter that cause the problem. Frankly, we never evolved to be massive meat eaters. It was an occasional addition to the diet rather than the mainstay.

8. I never take time to plan meals for the coming week
You plan not to plan. Make a great decision to get ahead of the game by planning just once for the whole week. It only takes a few minutes and puts you firmly back in control of the entire food consumption process.

9. When I buy snack foods, I eat until I have finished the whole package.

Stop buying sugary snack foods. Eliminate the temptation. Ban them from your home, your work and from your life. Forever.

10. I eat for comfort.

But it never works, does it? Because we eat garbage for comfort. Break out the healthy snacks and chew on something that will enhance your wellbeing rather than destroy you from within.

11. I am a Snacker.

No problem. There are countless healthy snacks for you to enjoy. As your body celebrates your better diet, you won't mind snacking on healthy food because it's helping you achieve your best possible shape and health.

12. I don't count fat grams

Me neither. I just avoid processed fats and sugars so the arithmetic is never a challenge.

13. I eat cookies, candy bars, or ice cream in place of dinner.

You're in trouble. These foods are slowly poisoning you. You're going to have to go cold turkey, dump the bad food and start eating normally. I don't think half measures are the answer. Swear an oath of allegiance to your poor body and start supporting it with good nutrition before it quits on you. Now is an excellent moment to begin.

14. When I don't plan meals, I eat fast food.

Planning is the key. Take a few minutes at the weekend to sketch out a meal plan for every day. One decision for the entire week. If it works for you, you can use it again and again. Tweak the plan. Add some variety. Enjoy being in control of your life and your health.

15. I eat when I am upset.

The long term answer is to learn not to be so easily upset but, in the meantime, choosing a healthy food that will fill you up without costing years of ill health makes a lot more sense than stuffing yourself with toxic waste.

16. I buy meat every time I go to the grocery store.

Lean, organic meat is the only alternative for the dedicated carnivore. It is vital to avoid the mass produced flesh that is full of antibiotics, hormones and fat.

17. I snack more at night.

It's another of those important house rules. Nothing to eat after eight in the evening except raw vegetables. Period.

18. I rarely eat breakfast.

Skipping breakfast ruins your day and sets you up for those nasty, unhealthy snacks that you use to keep you going. A healthy breakfast is the only way to start the day, kick start the metabolism and give your body the power to tackle everything that needs to be done. Sometimes it's just a question of making a simple plan for breakfast and being organised enough to make time for it.

19. I don't try to limit the intake of red meat (beef).

You can have too much of a good thing, even pure, organic beef. We simply didn't evolve to consume vast quantities of red meat every day. Hunting didn't allow for such a rich diet. Choose a couple of days per week when you can really enjoy your beef and remember that even the leanest beef is forty percent fat.

20. When I am in a bad mood, I eat whatever I feel like eating.

Sometimes a bad mood makes us feel guilty and that's when we choose self-destructive behaviour. If you choose food that's harmful for you, you're going to feel worse. It won't just be your mood that's causing you pain. Your body will feel awful too. That's what happens when you abuse it.

21. I never know what I am going to eat for supper when I get up in the morning.

When you take a few minutes to set up a fool proof eating plan for the entire week, you'll know exactly what you're going to eat. Because you already planned it. So tick that item off your To Do list. It's taken care of.

22. I never snack two to three times a day.

Much depends on how active you are during the day and what kind of work you're doing. If you're burning the calories, especially if you add exercise workouts to your routine, healthy snacks are a perfect supplement to your eating requirements. Healthy snacks are the perfect antidote to sugary toxic snacks.

23. Fish and poultry are the only meats I don't eat.

In my experience, the problem here is usually related to how the food is prepared. A good recipe and a little creativity can transform most fish and poultry into a feast. It's a great excuse to experiment!

24. When I am upset, I tend to eat more

And then you feel worse. We encourage absolutely everyone to learn to breathe more deeply, practise a little gentle meditation and distance yourself from the old habits of being upset. Food is often used as a drug. You use it as an escape mechanism. You use it as a displacement activity. If you need to chew, hit the raw veggies and you may find your mood as well as your health improves.

25. I like to eat vegetables seasoned with fatty meat.

Because it tastes good? Yep! And you crave the comfort of fat. Switch to virgin olive oil and save that fatty meat for the cat.

26. If I eat a larger than usual lunch, I won't skip supper.

Skipping meals is rarely a good idea. It's fine to have supper but make sure it's a smaller serving than usual.

27. I never take a shopping list to the grocery store.

Humans can't handle too many items of information at one time. That's why we invented lists. Then you don't have to try to remember everything you need at the store. Everything is on the list. It's called preparation and it makes life so much easier. Try it and see.

28. If I am bored, I will snack more

Boredom is a sure sign of an idle intelligence. We are surrounded by more visual stimulation, electronic media and entertainment material than at any other time in the history of the species and you're bored? Are you still alive? Wake up and open your eyes. The world around you is a miracle. Experience it every single day. And you are part of it.

29. I eat whatever I want at social events.
You have to be prepared. Once you begin to understand the real consequences of poisoning your body - and there's no pretty way of describing this - you'll take full responsibility for what goes into the cake hole. Putting your body under strain with toxic food can trigger problems that can kill you. Social events are meant to be enjoyed. They're not supposed to be lethal.

30. I am not very conscious of how much fat is in the food I eat.
We live in a world where this information is now widely available. As you develop awareness of what to eat, you'll find yourself checking labels more often. Getting in shape is a very important part of boosting good health and confidence. Keeping in good shape just requires a little more awareness. No more chomping like a zombie. Wake up and start paying attention to the things that can either help or harm. And that applies to what you eat.

31. I usually keep cookies in the house.
House rules! Make it a cast iron, non-negotiable rule - no cookies in the house. No junk food in the house. Scrap the temptation and you won't have to fight the urge to poison yourself.

32. I have a serving of meat at every meal.
Don't you get bored with meat? Don't you need some variety in your diet? Times have changed. The developed world has never had such incredible access to a truly vast array of foodstuffs. Give your taste buds a treat and your health a boost by enjoying delicious, nutritious food every single day/

33. I associate success with food.
There's a definite shift in cultural expectations. We used to associate success with cigars, alcohol and rich, sugary foods. Now we know better. Success also means feeling great, respecting the miracle of your body and living a healthy life so that you can enjoy the success. It's only a question of habits. You can easily associate success with getting a massage, enjoying a really healthy meal, taking better care of yourself. That's total success.

34. A complete meal includes a meat, a starch, a vegetable and bread.
It's amazing that these medieval ideas can persist for so long when the world is full of new data, new perspectives and life changing research. If you've been following the advice in your workbook you'll know pretty well what you need to eat and what to avoid to get into the best possible shape and discover the joys of real health.

35. On Sunday, I eat a large meal with my family.
What a perfect opportunity to share the good news about healthy nutrition and respecting your body. Be the example to your family. Be the change that motivates them to take care of themselves. Share your new knowledge. Spread the word. They only get the one life. Help them to make the very most of it by encouraging them to join you in a total commitment to feeling fantastic.

36. Instead of planning meals, I will replace supper with a snack.
Make it a house rule. Three healthy meals a day and healthy snacks to keep your appetite under control.

37. If I am busy, I will eat a snack instead of lunch.

Everyone's busy. How come some people get a healthy lunch? They prepare in advance. Organisation is the answer. Start planning for great things in your life, including great nutrition.

38. Sometimes I eat dessert more than once a day.

Sugar will kill you. You know that. You're giving yourself nasty insulin spikes with those desserts. The only way to handle the addiction is to go cold turkey and ban sugar for three days. That's how long it takes for your insulin levels to reset. Then it gets much, much easier.

39. To me, cookies or crunchy food are an ideal snack food.

Poison is never ideal unless you want to die. Slowly. Sugar is toxic. How can a toxic substance make you feel well? It doesn't, does it? Ban all cookies. Sugary crunchy snacks should have a skull and crossbones on the label. Ban the sugary snacks. The rule for living longer and enjoying your life is to banish sugar and anything that contains it.

40. My eating habits are very routine.

Fantastic! As long as you've developed the habits of eating healthily. If not, it's time to change those habits before your body starts to protest under the constant, habitual burden of food toxicity.

41. When choosing fast food, I pick a place that offers the tastes I like and not healthy foods.

Educating your palate can be tremendous fun but most of the foods we think we like are just an excuse to cram our guts with garbage. Might be healthier for you to save some money and dine right out of the dumpster. It's the sugar addiction - it's in so many foods these days that you're addicted to the stuff. Ban sugar from your diet and everything starts to get better. Stop poisoning yourself with garbage and start to appreciate what your body really needs.

42. I eat at a restaurant at least three times a week.

Eating out can be great fun. You just have to choose a restaurant with healthy food on the menu or ask the kitchen to make things for you that support your new wellbeing and health programme.

Summary - Getting organised

Identify your behaviours and eating choices

Learn to understand the real consequences of your behaviours

Accept your body and start to treat yourself with kindness and understanding

Identify where your habits and behaviours came from

Set up house rules and meal planning schedules

Switch on your awareness

I suggest taking a look at my Emotional Eating Book to further assist you in this area

Just search over the internet

www.amazon.com/gp/product/B00UZP82QO?ie=UTF8&camp=1789&creativeASIN=B00UZP82QO&linkCode=xm2&tag=onelifeblog-20

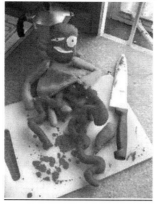

Chapter 6

Epigenetic GUT BIOLOGY

Your gut biology and the secrets of effective, sustained weight loss

Let's get right down to the guts of the matter! Whilst countless diet books have focused on fads and fleeting feeding fashions, we've had to wait until now to discover that the key to successful weight control is hidden in our intestinal flora. Encouraging the right balance of microbes in our gut and enhancing natural digestion are two of the most important and positive contributions we can make towards generating great health and real weight control.

There is an ancient tradition in many cultures that our intelligence is not simply located in the brain. You might find it surprising that recent research is taking a fresh look at this unusual question and producing some unexpected answers.

Dr Natasha Campbell McBride, an authority in this fascinating area, states "The importance of your gut flora, and its influence on your health cannot be overstated. It is truly profound. Your gut literally serves as your second brain and even produces more of the neurotransmitter serotonin - known to have a beneficial influence on your mood - than your brain does".

It gets better.

Your gut is also home to countless bacteria, both good and bad. These bacteria outnumber the cells in your body by at least ten to one. We refer to the world of your intestinal flora as the microbiome.

Your microbiome is closely inter-connected with both of your brain systems. Yes. We're proceeding on the basis that we have two locations for the body's operating systems. In addition to the brain in your head, embedded in the wall of your gut is the enteric nervous system (ENS), which works both independently of and in conjunction with the brain in your head.

According to New Scientist: "The ENS is part of the autonomic nervous system, the network of peripheral nerves that control visceral functions. It is also the original nervous system, emerging in the first vertebrates over 500 million years ago and becoming more complex as vertebrates evolved, possibly even giving rise to the brain itself."

Our ancient enteric nervous system is thought to be largely responsible for your "gut instincts," responding to environmental threats and sending information to your brain that directly affects your well-being. I'm sure you've experienced various sensations in your gut that accompany strong emotions such as fear, excitement and stress. Feeling "butterflies" in your stomach is actually the result of blood being diverted away from your gut to your muscles, as part of the fight or flight response.

These reactions in your gut happen outside of your conscious awareness because they are part of your autonomic nervous system, just like the beating of your heart. Your ENS contains around 500 million neurons. Why so many? Because eating is potentially fraught with danger: "Like the skin, the gut must stop potentially dangerous invaders, such as bacteria and viruses, from getting inside the body". This sounds like a perfectly helpful defence mechanism to foster our survival. And what better place to locate a defensive system to protect the body than in the very spot where food can cause the most damage: the gut.

Evolution really has been generous in equipping us with so many ways to keep us safe. If a pathogen should cross the gut lining, immune cells in the gut wall secrete inflammatory substances, including histamine, which are detected by neurons in the ENS. The gut brain then either triggers diarrhoea or alerts the brain in the head, which may decide to initiate vomiting, or both. In other words, the reactions in the gut will send instructions to purge the system as rapidly as possible.

We now know that this communication link between your "two brains" runs in both directions and is the main pathway for the way that foods affect your mood. For example, fatty foods make you feel good because fatty acids are detected by cell receptors in the lining of your gut, which then send warm and fuzzy nerve signals to your brain. Knowing this, you can begin to understand how not only your physical health but also your mental health is deeply influenced by the state of your gut and the microbial zoo that lives there. Your intestinal microbes affect your overall brain function, so this means that your eating behaviour is also affected by the health of your gut!

When it comes to Inflammation, Your Microbiome Rules

Scientists have found a specific pattern of intestinal microbes that can measurably increase your risk for Type 2 diabetes. This pattern can serve as a biomarker for diabetes probability. Similarly, researchers have also found marked differences in bacterial strains between overweight and non-overweight people. A strain of beneficial bacteria called Lactobacillus rhamnosus has been identified as being helpful for women to lose weight.

The best way to optimize your gut flora is through your diet. A gut-healthy diet is one rich in whole, unprocessed, unsweetened foods, along with traditionally fermented or cultured foods. But before these powerful foods can work their magic in your body, you have to eliminate the damaging foods that get in their way.

The conclusions of the latest research confirm that a good place to start is by drastically reducing grains and sugar. We covered this in our very first piece of advice. Did you print out the warning and tape it to your fridge? We also need to avoid genetically engineered ingredients, processed foods, and pasteurised foods. Pasteurised foods can harm your good bacteria and sugar promotes the growth of pathogenic yeast and other fungi (not to mention fuelling cancer cells). Grains containing gluten are particularly damaging to your microflora and overall health. This would be a good time for you to review the table above that lists foods, drugs and other agents that harm your beneficial microbes so that you can take steps right now to avoid as many as possible.

And In with the Good!

Consuming naturally fermented foods is one of the best ways to optimize your microbiome.

Not only are your gut bacteria important for preventing disease, but they also play a critical role in defining your body weight and composition.

Scientific studies have revealed a positive-feedback loop between the foods you crave and the composition of your microbiome, which depends on those nutrients for survival. So, if you're craving sugar and refined carbohydrates, you may actually be feeding a voracious army of Candida! Once you've begun eliminating foods that damage your beneficial flora, start incorporating fermented foods such as sauerkraut and naturally fermented pickles for example.

Your gut bacteria - and therefore your physical and mental health - are continuously affected by your environment, and by your diet and lifestyle choices. If your microbiome is harmed and thrown out of balance (dysbiosis), all sorts of illnesses can result, both acute and chronic. Unfortunately, your fragile internal ecosystem is under constant assault nearly every single day.

Some of the factors posing the gravest dangers to your microbiome are outlined in the following table. You should be already familiar with some of these toxic substances from previous chapters!

- Refined sugar, especially processed high fructose corn syrup (HFCS)
- Genetically engineered (GE) foods (extremely abundant in processed foods and beverages)
- Agricultural chemicals, such as herbicides and pesticides. Glyphosate appears to be among the worst
- Conventionally-raised meats and other animal products; CAFO animals are routinely fed low-dose antibiotics and GE livestock are raised on Gluten
- Antibiotics (use only if absolutely necessary, and make sure to reseed your gut with fermented foods and/or a good probiotic supplement) NSAIDs (Nonsteroidal anti-inflammatory drugs) damage cell membranes and disrupt energy production by mitochondria)

The microbes in our gut have evolved to function as highly efficient food processors and they are directly affected by whatever we eat. When the microbiome is out of balance, we often see varying degrees of inflammation throughout the body.

The Epigenetic Eating Program, which is blissfully free of refined grains, flour, sugar, and processed vegetable oils supports the healthiest mixture of gut microflora. On the other hand, the typical Western diet – very high in calories from refined carbohydrates but lacking in essential nutrients – tends to have the opposite effect, contributing to a harmful imbalance in gut bacteria. This is so serious that it can lead to the development of insulin resistance, diabetes, obesity, and heart disease. An unhealthy microbiome naturally tends towards weight gain so we can see how closely our health and wellbeing is linked to the state of our intestinal flora. When the unhealthy microbes predominate in the gut, they send signals to the brain to supply more fuel in the form of refined carbohydrates, dramatically increasing the chances of you putting on more weight. As we've stated earlier in the book, taking control of your weight is only one of the benefits of creating a normal and healthy environment for your gut flora. Better health, longer life and a reduction in the risk of disease are all connected to a healthy, efficient and happy microbiome!

Gut Biology Summary

The gut is the site of the 'second brain'

Inflammatory conditions are deeply influenced by the microbiome

Correcting intestinal flora is the key to health and weight loss

Identify the toxins that harm the body and disrupt normal gut functioning

Eliminate harmful substances from daily diet to restore balance

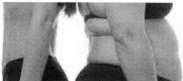

Chapter 7

YOUR ANTI INFLAMMATORY Paleo – Keto - Epigenetic Eating Transformation

Welcome to Your brand new and exciting career! You are now Managing Director of Your Paleo-Keto Epigenetic Eating Life. Inc. Congratulations. It's simply the Best Job in the Whole World and now it's yours.

Your most important job from now on is to focus on making the right food choices. You don't need to weigh or measure, you don't need to count calories. Wow, I bet that sounds like a new way of dealing with the old weight loss issue, doesn't it? Just make that one decision to follow the programme under any and all circumstances, under any amount of stress and your body will do the rest.

Your only job?

The most important job in your life!

Eat The Right Food for Your Epigenetic Expression

Fall madly in love with your absolute best weight-loss foods - and watch them fall in love with you and your new, leaner body

From all the information you've absorbed so far, you'll know for sure that certain food groups (like sugars, grains and dairy products) could be having a very negative impact on your health and wellbeing without you even noticing. But when you think about your present state of wellbeing, you might be wondering how much of your health - or lack of it - has been caused by the food you've been eating. Weight loss is a great example. If you've tried to lose weight but always found it a struggle, experiencing initial success but then putting the pounds back on, you know that you have to do something different. It's time to recognise that cutting down the calories isn't enough. If you're still eating the wrong foods, the problems will remain. It's time to remove the source of the problem and that's only going to happen by removing all the harmful, toxic foods from your diet.

Say goodbye to all the psychologically unhealthy, hormone-unbalancing, gut-disrupting, inflammatory food groups and see the weight fall off. That's right. You might want to read that sentence again. It's essential to your future health. Let your body heal and recover from the years and years of weight gain and from all the other nasty effects of those nasty, toxic foods. It's time to re-programme your metabolism and flush away the inflammation.

FIGHTING FIBROMYALGIA With THE ANTI- INFLAMMATORY DIET By Mercedes Del Rey

Learn once and for all how the foods you've been eating are really affecting your health, your weight and your long term health. We've arrived at one of the most important reasons for you to follow this programme.

This is about to change your life.

Epigenetics demonstrates the vital link between the things you do and how you live to the way your body behaves, all the way down to the cellular level. This might be one of the most surprising revelations about the entire body transformation programme. I think you're going to like it because you're going to love the results.

We cannot possibly put enough emphasis on this simple fact.

Like many of the most important elements in our lives, the answers are so simple that it's too easy to blink and miss the power of this revelation.

The Epigenetic Eating Transformation

Are you ready for this?

Well, take a deep breath, my friend, because this is the answer you've been waiting for.

Eat. Real. Food.

Eat real food.

Only eat real food.

And now you know.

Real food is unprocessed, additive free and as natural as nature intended.

Real food includes lean, organic game and poultry, line caught seafood, organic free range eggs, tons of fresh vegetables, some fruit, and plenty of good fats from fruits, oils, nuts and seeds.

Eat foods with very few ingredients and no additives, chemicals, sugars or flavourings. Better yet, eat foods with no ingredients listed at all because then they're totally natural and unprocessed.

Don't worry, these guidelines are outlined in extensive detail in our essential life-enhancing Epigenetic Eating Shopping list.

What to avoid if you want to be healthier, leaner and in better shape forever.

More importantly, here's what NOT to eat. Cutting out all of these foods and drinks will help you regain your natural, healthy metabolism, reduce systemic inflammation and help you to realise exactly how these foods are truly affecting your weight, fat percentage, health, fitness and every aspect of your life.

- Sugar. It's out. It's that simple. Do not consume added sugar of any kind whether it's real or artificial. No maple syrup, honey, agave nectar, coconut sugar, Splenda, Equal, Nutrasweet, Xylitol. The only exception is Stevia, the natural sweetener that avoids the toxicity of all the other sweeteners. Start reading the labels because food companies love to use sugar in their products to cater for your sugar addiction and they use it in ways you might not recognise. Great way to sell more products. Disastrous for your health.
- Do not consume beer in any form, not even for cooking. And let's be brutal about that other global addiction - tobacco. Absolutely no tobacco products of any sort. Ever. Wine though, in moderation, is fine. Ideally you'll opt for dry wines and a small amount of spirits but NO liqueurs ever!
- Do not eat grains. This includes wheat, rye, barley, oats, corn, rice, millet, bulgur, or sprouted grains
- The very occasional exceptions are buckwheat and quinoa which are not technically grains but, unfortunately, they have many grain like qualities. The answer is to limit your consumption and always

exercise moderation. Cutting out grains also includes all the ways we add wheat, corn, rice and other starches to our foods in the form of bran, wheat germ, modified starch and so on. Again, read the labels.

- Do not eat legumes, except for some occasional sprouted legumes. This includes beans of all kinds (black, red, pinto, navy, white, kidney, lima, fava, etc.), peas, chickpeas, lentils, and peanuts. No peanut butter, either. This also includes all forms of soy, soy sauce, miso, tofu, tempeh, edamame and all the many ways we sneak soy into foods (like lecithin).
- Do not eat dairy. This includes cow, goat or sheep's milk and milk products such as cream, cheese (hard or soft), kefir, yogurt (even Greek), and sour cream. Use coconut milk, coconut yoghurt and coconut cream.
- Do not consume carrageenan, MSG, sulphites or any additives whatsoever. If these ingredients or any E numbers appear in any form on the label of your processed food or beverage, don't even touch it!.

Sounds tough, doesn't it? But that's because we've been conditioned to connect really bad food and sugary sweet flavourings with good times. We get sweets and candy as a reward during childhood and the comforting feeling gets embedded in our behaviour.

Before long we're addicted to all the things that effectively poison us. Take a look around you. Do you see much evidence of happy, healthy people in the local population? Disease incidence and obesity are ballooning. Something's radically wrong and you are one of the few, lucky ones to know exactly where the problem really lies.

Knowledge is power, my friend. Let's put this life-changing knowledge to the best possible use. Right now. You know what to do. All you have to do is make one powerful choice for health, normal weight and a tremendous increase in energy and the quality of your life and your body will do the rest.

At this stage of the programme, you might be surprised to know that we're not going to obsess too much about the weighting scales. The really important changes are taking place inside your body and your weight will improve naturally as you allow it to flush out all the toxins and reduce inflammation levels.

The Fine Print

These foods are the exceptions to the rule and the good news is they are all allowed in your new super healthy eating plan

- Certain legumes. Green beans and peas. While they're technically a legume, these are generally good for you.
- Vinegar. Most forms of vinegar, including white, apple cider, red wine, and rice, are allowed. The only exceptions are balsamic, vinegars with added sugar, or malt vinegar, which generally contains gluten.

- Salt but only low sodium or sodium-free salt. Did you know that all iodised table salt contains sugar? Sugar (often in the form of dextrose) is chemically essential to keep the potassium iodide from oxidising and being lost.

Limitation Foods – be careful 5%

High sugar fruits – watermelon, grapes, mangoes.

Buckwheat and quinoa – it behaves like a starchy carbohydrate a bit

Clever but slightly naughty indulgences – 10%

Chocolate – organic cocoa powder,

Fried potatoes – use sweet potatoes or lots of vinegar to help with digestion,

Muffins cakes and cookies with almond and coconut flour and stevia

Nut and Seed Butters. Its ok but still processed

Fats to help you burn fat – 20--%

Coconut oil, extra virgin olive oil, walnuts, macadamias and their oils, coconut products, avocados

Vegetables to fuel your system 30%

Really go to town and enjoy as many servings in as many formats as you can...raw is best, but steamed and stir fried work wonderfully well

Proteins for weight loss 35%

Fish, Turkey (chicken if you must), game and hemp seed protein are the best forms for weight loss

The PALEO/KETO Epigenetic Shopping Guide

Being overweight is expensive in every possible way. And it costs far too much in terms of your quality of life. So it's vitally important to make healthy eating your absolute top priority and there are many of ways for you to maximize your food budget. We'll start with the top foods in the PALEO/KETO Epigenetic Eating Diet

The next three items ALL SHARE EQUAL PRIORITY

#1: Protein

Always start at the game, poultry, fish, and eggs section first because the majority of your budget should be spent on high quality animal protein.

- Prime choice:

Always look for organic and/or raised in the wild. Buy whatever's available, and learn how to cook it, if necessary. If you have room in your budget, buy extra and freeze it for later. Go for organic, free-range eggs – they're still one of the cheapest sources of good protein.

- Alternative choice:

If you can't afford organic meat, go for game (ostrich and venison are best), fish and eggs. Chicken is still controversial because we don't know how many hormones and GMO grains are added to chickenfeed these days. Avoid beef and pork since they are too high in fat and usually contain anti-biotics and hormones.

- Never:

Bypass all commercially-raised and/or processed meats (like bacon, sausage and deli meats).

- If you are against consuming animal protein for any reason, you have a great alternative in Hemp Protein Powder

Hemp protein, made from the hemp seed, is a high-fibre protein supplement that can be used to enhance total protein intake for vegans and non-vegans alike. Hemp can be considered a superior protein source due to its above-average digestibility, which also makes it ideal for athletes. When a protein is efficiently digested, it can be deployed more effectively by the body. The digestibility of any given protein is related to the concentrations of its amino acids. A study published in 2010 in the "Journal of Agricultural and Food Chemistry" tested the protein digestibility-corrected amino acid score (PDAAS) -- a rating that determines the bioavailability of a protein -- for various proteins derived from the hemp seed. The results showed that hemp seed proteins have PDAAS values greater than or equal to a variety of grains, nuts and legumes. We're big fans of hemp seed protein because it enhances the immune system and boosts energy levels as well as protecting the kidneys.

Hemp Background

Hemp is a remarkably diverse crop that can be grown for both food and non-food purposes. Hemp seed, which is used to manufacture hemp protein, is composed of approximately 45 percent oil, 35 percent protein and 10 percent carbohydrates. The hemp seed possesses many nutritional benefits, according to Agriculture and Agri-food Canada. In addition to its health benefits, hemp is very environmentally friendly, as it can be grown without the use of fungicides, herbicides and pesticides and it efficiently absorbs carbon dioxide. How many more good reasons do you need to fall in love with hemp seed protein?

#2: Vegetables

Now that you've organised your essential protein supplies, it's time to move on to the vegetables. These are the second tier of your super new plan for effective weight loss and new levels of wellbeing.

- Vegetables are very important in the epigenetic diet plan because they help the body to eliminate toxins and re-balance the microbiome. (By this we mean your gut bacteria). Local produce is the first choice and aim to eat whatever's in season as these veggies are going to be the least expensive and the most nutritious. Choose veggies that are super dense with nutrients. If you have to peel it before eating (or if you don't eat the skin), organic isn't as important. Frozen vegetables can also be an excellent budget-friendly option.
- Fruits: Buy what you can locally (and organically, if possible). If you can't get it locally then it's probably not in season, which means it's not as fresh, not as tasty, and more expensive. Frozen fruits (like berries) are superb, inexpensive alternatives. Add berries and low sugar apples to your shopping list. Bananas, peaches and pineapple should always be consumed in very small quantities and we recommend that you avoid during detox grapes, mango, tropical and dried fruit especially during the three week detox phase….after that always eat sparingly.

#3: Healthy Fats

Healthy fats make up the last but most important item on your shopping list. Some of the healthiest fats are also the least expensive and it's always a good idea to keep a good supply of oils, nuts, and seeds at home to help in preparing your super, new Epigenetic meals.

- Canned coconut milk is delicious and provides 72 grams of fat per can. Avocados are a great, all year-round choice too when it comes to sourcing healthy fat.
- Almond milk and other nut-based milks are also recommended but always make sure there is no sugar or salt in the list of ingredients
- Almond or coconut flour make an ideal alternative for baking or for thickening sauces.
- Stock up on coconut oil, extra virgin olive oil, walnut, avocado and hazelnut oil.
- Nuts are a great source of healthy fats but you need to consume them in moderation. Nut butters often contain unnecessary additives to be careful to read the labels. Too many cheaper nuts are salted and roasted in seed or vegetable oils – a less healthy option – so always opt for the raw, natural varieties.

Additional Items

Low Sodium Salt – An Absolute Essential

Let's start with the fact that sodium is an essential part of your daily diet. But, as many of us now know, too much sodium can be downright harmful to the body. Lower levels of sodium in the diet can really help your heart, kidneys, and all of your body systems.. The 2010 Dietary Guidelines for Americans recorded by the MayoClinic.com recommends that adults who are healthy should limit sodium to no more than 2,300 mg/day.

Sodium and Your Health

Cut down your salt intake.

The American Heart Association states that "Sodium is an element that's needed for good health. However, too much salt or too much water in your system will upset the balance." There are many benefits to following a low sodium diet. Reducing your intake of sodium, or salt, helps to reduce blood pressure and helps to prevent swelling of the extremities, such as your legs.

People who reduce their salt intake may experience an initial weight loss that is rapid, but limited. Sodium causes a person to retain water, which adds to body weight, according to Diets in Review, an online resource about healthy eating. Though someone who begins a low-sodium diet may be pleasantly surprised to see a seemingly large weight loss at first, these results typically end once the dieter returns to adding the more usual amounts of salt to their daily eating habits.

Important Considerations

Not all stevia is the same. Do try several different brands but always ensure that there are no other additives whatsoever. Stevia liquid in glycerite tends to be the best tasting!

Ways to Reduce Sodium

Salt often disguises the more subtle flavours in our food so it can be a very pleasant surprise to banish salt and discover what real food tastes like! Checking food labels will soon reveal how many daily products contain added salt. It's everywhere,.. Frozen dinners, for example, can have low fat content but very high sodium levels. Using fresh or frozen vegetables can help reduce the sodium content of foods, and rinsing canned vegetables can rid them of the salt that is used in the preservation process. Using fresh or dried herbs can give meat, fish and vegetables a fabulous flavour without adding salt, fat or calories. Once you get used to less salt in your food, your taste buds come alive and reward you with a whole new sensory experience with layers of delightful subtlety that can revolutionise the eating experience forever.

The only safe sweetener for Weight Loss

Using the highly refined extracts from the stevia leaf as a zero-calorie, 100 percent natural sweetener can help reduce your intake of sugar. Stevia is actually 300 times sweeter than regular sugar with a minimal aftertaste, yet it is suitable for sugar-sensitive people, such as diabetics. Stevia will not cause cavities and is heat-resistant enough for use in baking and cooking, according to the 2005 book by; Dr. Gillian McKeith called Living Food for Health. Refined, simple sugars are a leading cause of obesity in the U.S., according to KidsHealth, and substituting other non-caloric sweeteners for table sugar can promote weight loss and maintenance.

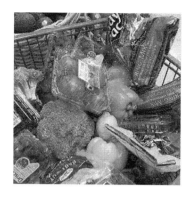

The ANTI INFLAMMATORY Paleo-Keto Epigenetic Delicious Shopping List

Items in *italics* – limit choice

PROTEIN:

Seafood

Not Good	: Farm-raised
Better	: Organic
Best	: Wild-caught & sustainably fished

Poultry

Not Good	: Factory farmed
Better	: Free-Range
Best	: Organic

Game

Not Good	: Processed Game Products

Better   : Wild-caught

Best   : 100% grass-fed & organic

Eggs

Not Good   : Factory farmed

Better   : (omega-3 enriched optional)

Best   : organic

VEGETABLES:

Acorn Squash

Fennel Root

Artichoke

Arugula

Asparagus

Beets

Bell Peppers

Bok Choy

Broccoli/baby broccoli

Brussels Sprouts

Butternut Squash

Cabbage

Carrots

Cauliflower

Celery

Cucumber

Eggplant

Garlic

Green Beans

Greens (beet, mustard, turnip)

Kale

Leeks

Lettuce (butter, red)

Mushrooms (all)

Okra

Onion/Shallots

Parsnips

Potatoes – smaller red skinned are ideal-limit consumption to very moderate

Pumpkin

Radish

Rhubarb

Snow/Sugar Snap Peas

Spaghetti Squash

Spinach

Sprouts

Summer Squash

Sweet Potato/Yams

Swiss Chard

Tomato

Turnip

Watercress

Zucchini - Courgettes

FRUITS: BEST FOR PALEO-KETO

Blackberries

Blueberries

Cherries

Grapefruit

Kiwi

Lemon/Lime

Nectarines

Papaya

Peaches

Plum

Pomegranate

Raspberries

Strawberries

Tangerines

NO DRIED FRUIT

FATS

Best: Cooking Fats

Coconut oil

Extra-Virgin Olive Oil

Best: Eating Fats

Avocado

Cashews

Coconut Butter

Coconut Meat/Flakes

Coconut Milk (canned)

Hazelnuts/Filberts

Macadamia Nuts

Macadamia Butter

Nuts and Seeds

Almonds

Almond Butter

Brazil Nuts

Pecans

Pistachio

Flax Seeds

Pine Nuts

Pumpkin Seeds

Sesame Seeds

Sunflower Seeds

Seed Butters

Walnuts

Summary

Fall in love with the best weight-loss foods

Eliminate sugars, grains and dairy products from your diet

Eat real, natural, unprocessed food

Eliminate additives

Eliminate legumes

Take charge of your body, your weight and your well being

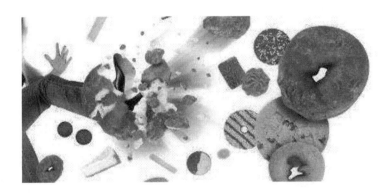

Chapter 8

Toxins and genetic interference – causing inflammation and weight loss problems

Food processing or food poisoning techniques?

The modern industrial approach to food production and processing is responsible for a ghastly range of chemicals and additives that are directly involved in producing weight gain, fat and obesity. Amongst the thousands of additives, we have bovine growth hormone and antibiotics injected into meat, poultry, and dairy products, flavour enhancers such as monosodium glutamate, artificial sweeteners such as NutraSweet (aspartame) and Splenda (sucralose). Our list also includes man-made sugars such as high fructose corn syrup, corn syrup, dextrose, sucrose, fructose, highly refined white sugar, processed molasses, processed honey, maltodextrin, etc., plus the other 15,000 plus chemicals that are routinely added to virtually every product you buy, and that includes conventionally grown fruits and vegetables.

Man-made trans-fats such as hydrogenated or partially hydrogenated oils also cause weight gain and obesity. Even standard food processing techniques such as pasteurisation, which now applies to virtually every product in a bottle or carton, homogenisation and irradiation all contribute to weight gain.

At the end of this disturbing list of toxins, poisons and health-damaging additives we have some refreshing and deeply reassuring news. Your revolutionary epigenetic weight control system addresses all of these issues safely and effectively and offers the fast lane out of the nightmare of processed food. Once you know you have the tools to make things better, you can breathe a sigh of relief and start to take action..

Poisons polluting the planet and everything that lives on it. You've probably heard a lot already about the increasing levels of toxicity in the environment. The fact is that our environment has become increasingly more toxic. Our exposure today is higher than at any point in human history.

We are exposed to more than 10,000 different forms of toxin and they are almost everywhere. They're in the air we breathe, the water we drink and wash in, our daily cleaning materials, cosmetics and, of course, our precious food supplies. If you add the daily quota of toxic chemicals we consume in the form of artificial sweeteners, flavour enhancers such as MSG, pesticides, preservatives, caffeine, over-the-counter medications, alcohol, nicotine and damaged fats, the list of daily toxic consumption could give you nightmares. But beyond the discomfort of a nightmare, these toxins are harming your body. We should also include those naturally occurring toxins produced by the body as a result of normal, essential cellular functions.

The problem is that these pesky toxins can accumulate in the body and that's when the damage occurs. It is the accumulation of these toxins that creates total havoc in the body. Yes we can process and remove many harmful substances and neutralise their influence but when we take on board more than we can handle, the body is effectively poisoned. As a result, excessive oxidative stress occurs, which in turn threatens our health by damaging our precious DNA. And as you now know, damaged DNA can lead to a long list of health problems.

Let's get this uncomfortable subject sharply into focus. Entire populations are suffering the effects of toxicity: the problems show up as a combination of headaches, fatigue, joint pain, insomnia, mood changes, weakened immune system, or other chronic issues. This total toxic overload has been implicated in: cardiovascular disease, cancer, chronic fatigue, weight loss resistance, allergies, skin conditions, asthma, mental illness, hypertension, gastritis, kidney disease and obesity. Not a happy list.

We know you like to have all the facts so let's see how toxins can even influence human metabolism.

There are five important mechanisms that are harmed by toxins:

Hormone regulation,

Neuro-regulatory mechanisms,

Immuno-regulatory mechanisms,

Mitochondrial function,

And oxidative stress.

Toxins alter thyroid hormone metabolism and receptor function leading to a slow down in metabolic rate. Slower metabolic activity means more fat retention. It isn't difficult to see the connections between constant exposure to toxins and lots of nasty little health problems, unintended weight gain being one of the most obvious.

The Environmental Protection Agency in the U.S. has monitored human exposure to toxic environmental chemicals since 1972.

That's when they began the National Human Adipose Tissue Survey. This study measures the levels of various toxins in fat tissue extracted during autopsies and from surgical procedures. Five of what are recognised as the most toxic chemicals were found in 100% of all samples.

Toxic chemicals from industrial pollution dominated the samples, toxins that damage the liver, heart, lungs, and nervous system. Nine more chemicals were found in 91-98% of samples: benzene, toluene, ethyl benzene, DDE (a breakdown product of DDT, the pesticide banned in the US since 1972), three dioxins, and one furan. Polychlorinated biphenyls (PCBs) were found in 83% of the population.

A Michigan study found DDT in over 70% of 4 years olds, probably received through breast milk. With the spread of the global economy, we may be eating food that was picked a few days before in Guatemala, Indonesia, Africa or Asia, where there are fewer restrictions on pesticides than there are in the United States or Europe.

I don't want to put you off your lunch but many of these chemicals are stored in fat tissue, making animal products a potentially concentrated source of contamination. One hundred percent of beef in the U.S. is contaminated with DDT, as is 93% of processed cheese, hot dogs, bologna, turkey, and ice cream. Bon appetit!

But just because there are plenty of reasons to get paranoid about our food, there are plenty of healthy, life-affirming, nourishing and tasty alternatives out there.

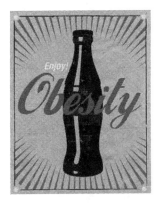

OBESITY, INFLAMMATION AND TOXICITY: What is the real connection?

Effects on Thyroid and Metabolic Rate

If you've ever attempted a weight loss programme, you'll probably recognise the familiar plateau phase where many people lose a few pounds but then find it really difficult to shed the rest.

What might be getting in the way of further weight loss and even interfering with the metabolic control system? A review paper, "Energy balance and pollution by organochlorines and polychlorinated biphenyls," published in Obesity Reviews in 2003 describes the effects of toxins on metabolic rate and weight regulation.

The authors conclude that pesticides (organochlorines) and PCBs (from industrial pollution), which are normally stored in fat tissue, are released during the weight loss process and lower the metabolic rate. That will slow down the rate at which we can lose the pounds. How do the chemical toxins interfere with our metabolism?

People with a higher body mass index (BMI) have a larger volume of places to hold onto the toxins. They store more toxins because they have more fat. Those toxins interfere with many normal aspects of metabolism, including reducing thyroid hormone levels, and increasing excretion of thyroid hormones via the liver.

Toxins also compete with the thyroid hormones by blocking the thyroid receptors and competing for the thyroid transport proteins. We all know that toxins are bad news for the health but clearly we need to have an effective strategy to deal with the effects of toxins leaking into the system as we launch our weight management system. The good news is that we've got a great strategy for handling this problem! And we'll be getting to it very soon.

The Secret Power of Leptin!

Leptin is a very powerful and influential hormone and it's produced by your fat cells.

Putting it simply, science has discovered that leptin is an incredibly powerful metabolic regulator and it tells your brain whether you should be hungry, whether you should eat and whether to produce more fat. Leptin is the way that your fat communicates with your brain to let your body know how much energy is available and, very importantly, what to do with it.

In a perfect world, as you gain weight, you secrete more leptin from your fat cells. This in turn tells your brain you have stored enough fat so it naturally reduces your appetite, sending messages to help you balance your system by burning excess fat.

But there's a problem! Sometimes the leptin doesn't get the chance to communicate effectively. It isn't good news because many people have something called "leptin resistance". This means that no matter how much leptin you create from your fat cells, the brain just doesn't see it. This leads to a cycle of unhappy consequences.

Your brain thinks you are starving, so you burn fewer calories, your appetite goes into overdrive and finally every morsel of food you consume gets stored around your belly! So, until you address leptin resistance, you're not going to lose weight.

Optimal Leptin Levels

When you have your leptin levels checked by a professional, your goal is to keep your leptin below 12. But not too low. Researchers have discovered that when leptin levels fall too far below the 12 mark, we can expect an increase in Alzheimer's and dementia. A leptin above 12 is not considered healthy either.

Leptin levels can now be measured with a simple blood test. Levels above 12 are linked to weight gain, accelerated ageing, increased risk of infertility, diabetes and heart attack. In addition, high leptin levels are associated with belly fat and numerous cancers. Leptin rises if you don't sleep well and if you have any kind of perceived stress. So it really is an important and often ignored component in the whole weight control mechanism.

Thyroid Connection

If you are having difficulty losing weight, I recommend you get your leptin checked. Remember you want it under 12. From a thyroid perspective, if your leptin is above 12 you will commonly see low T3 (the most metabolically active thyroid hormone) and elevated reverse T3. This is not good for those trying to lose weight.

The Solution:

You become leptin resistant by eating the typical American or western diet, which is full of sugar, refined grains, and processed foods. The solution is to eat a diet that emphasises good fats and avoids blood sugar spikes.

These answers are often surprising because they really are incredibly simple. When you choose a diet that emphasises those essential, healthy fats, lean meats and lots and lots of vegetables, (raw whenever possible), your body can recover its natural healthy functioning and those pesky pounds start to melt away,

For a full thyroid/leptin analysis, I recommend a medical practitioner with a thorough training and knowledge in functional medicine.

For a list of Functional Medicine Doctors in your area contact us via our website,

www.skinnydeliciouslife.com

Toxins Summary

Pollutions and toxins are everywhere

Obesity and toxicity are closely related

The power of leptins

The thyroid connection

Cleansing and healing the body for permanent weight control

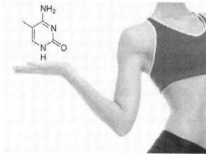

Chapter9

The Epigenetic Exercise Myth

The Epigenetics of Exercise

Far from being written in stone, genetic expression can be altered by influences coming from outside the gene. This influence alters the operation of the gene, but does not affect the DNA blueprint itself. This process is known as epigenetics.

Toxic exposure also tends to affect genetic expression, by altering the types of proteins a particular gene will express.

In this way, your environment, diet, and general lifestyle play a significant role in your state of health and development of disease. When it comes to exercise, previous research has found that exercise can induce *immediate* changes in the methylation patterns of genes found in your muscle cells.

Several of the genes affected by an acute bout of exercise are genes involved in fat metabolism. Specifically, the study suggests that when you exercise, your body almost immediately experiences genetic activation that increases the production of fat-busting proteins.

Quite clearly, exercise in all its forms tends to have a positive effect. It has the power to affect your entire body, and your overall state of health. Its beneficial impact on your insulin response (normalizing your glucose and insulin levels by optimizing insulin receptor sensitivity) is among the most important benefits of exercise, as insulin resistance is a factor in most chronic disease.

The Many Biological Effects of Exercise

Getting back to the effects of exercise in general, a number of biological effects occur when you work out. This includes changes in your:

- **Muscles**, which use glucose and ATP for contraction and movement. To create more ATP, your body needs extra oxygen, so breathing increases and your heart starts pumping more blood to your muscles. Without sufficient oxygen, lactic acid will form instead. Tiny tears in your muscles make them grow bigger and stronger as they heal.

- **Lungs**. As your muscles call for more oxygen (as much as 15 times more oxygen than when you're at rest), your breathing rate increases. Once the muscles surrounding your lungs cannot move any faster, you have reached what's called your VO2 max your maximum capacity of oxygen use. The higher your VO2 max, the fitter you are.

- **Heart**. As mentioned, your heart rate increases with physical activity to supply more oxygenated blood to your muscles. The fitter you are, the more efficiently your heart can do this, allowing you to work out longer and harder. As a side effect, this increased efficiency will also reduce your *resting* heart rate. Your blood pressure will also decrease as a result of new blood vessels forming.

- **Joints and bones**, as exercise can place as much as five or six times more than your body weight on them. Peak bone mass is achieved in adulthood and then begins a slow decline, but exercise can help you to maintain healthy bone mass as you get older. Weight-bearing exercise is actually one of the most effective remedies against osteoporosis, as your bones are very porous and soft, and as you get older your bones can easily become less dense and hence, more brittle -- especially if you are inactive.

Exercise Is Important for Optimal Brain Health, Too

Genetic changes occur here, too. The increased blood flow adapts your brain to turn different genes on or off, and many of these changes help protect against diseases such as Alzheimers and Parkinsons. A number of neurotransmitters are also triggered, such as endorphins, serotonin, dopamine, glutamate, and GABA. Some of these are well-known for their role in mood control. Not surprisingly, exercise is one of the most effective prevention and treatment strategies for depression. Exercise Leverages Other Healthy Lifestyle Changes

While diet accounts for about 80 percent of the health benefits you get from a healthy lifestyle, exercise is the ultimate leveraging agent that kicks all those benefits up a notch. The earlier you begin and the more consistent you are, the greater your long-term rewards, but its never too late to start. Even seniors can improve their physical and mental health.

Its strongly recommend to avoid sitting as much as possible, and making it a point to walk more every day. A fitness tracker can be very helpful for this. I suggest aiming for 7,000 to 10,000 steps per day, *in addition to* your regular fitness regimen, not in lieu of it. The research is clearly showing that prolonged sitting is an independent risk factor for chronic disease and increases your mortality risk from *all* causes. So standing up more and engaging in non-exercise movement as much as possible is just as important for optimal health as having a regular fitness regimen.

FIGHTING FIBROMYALGIA With THE ANTI- INFLAMMATORY DIET By Mercedes Del Rey

One of the great myths about weight loss is that all you have to do is burn more calories and everything will be absolutely fine. Clearly, from all the information we've studied and absorbed so far, we know this cannot be the whole story.

We know for a fact that people can lose weight by burning more calories. No question.

The problem is that it's rarely a permanent loss. As soon as you take a break from the routine, the pounds pile back on. And we're committed to a permanent and healthy weight adjustment that will benefit every aspect of your life. So let's remind ourselves that if we're going to take control of our weight, we need to change our metabolism. If we can encourage our metabolism to speed up, we'll burn our food more efficiently and encourage our bodies to burn fat.

Adding exercise to our routine can certainly help to speed up the weight loss programme but we're encouraging you to exercise because it really can improve the overall quality of your life. We want you to be fitter, stronger, leaner, more flexible and happier in the way your body works. Does that sound like a good idea? Do you want to live in a body that works the way Nature intended? It's a lot more fun than being trapped in an overweight, physically uncomfortable body that lacks the energy and stamina to enjoy life to the full.

When it comes to exercise, we're truly spoiled for choice. It seems that every time we turn on the TV there's a super-fit girl or boy bouncing up and down with the latest fitness fad, screaming at us to join the craze. But fitness is not about fashion. It isn't about gadgets and it isn't about trying to look like someone else. It's about feeling great and making the body as efficient as nature intended. Yes, we have to move the body to make it fitter but using exercise intelligently will serve our purposes better than blindly following the latest exercise in television fitness marketing.

The first question to raise in our quest for intelligent exercise is "What kind of exercise will help me lose excess fat and weight most efficiently?" The short answer, perhaps not surprisingly, is the kind of exercise that burns the most calories. But we need to burn calories in the most efficient manner possible for the longest period of time whilst encouraging an increase in metabolic rate. OK. Not such a short answer but even a simple question can offer important insights into what we're really seeking in terms of safe, intelligent exercise.

There is a common consensus that cardiovascular workouts are the best in terms of straightforward calorie burning but there is a growing realisation that interval workouts, where we switch between short bursts of high intensity effort followed by brief periods of less intense exercise, are one of the best ways to turn up the fat-burning mechanism. Interval training can raise your metabolic rate for up to four hours after a session, meaning you'll burn more calories even after the workout is over.

Easy? Well before you jump into your exercise shorts and slip on the Spandex leotard, we need to recognise that too many intense cardio sessions can harm your body, causing burn out, leaving you tired, low in energy, suffering strained joints and muscles and too exhausted to keep up the exercise programme. Less is sometimes more. Try using the higher intensity interval approach a couple of days a week and substitute a less intense endurance session for your other workouts. Endurance training means exercising at an intensity where you can still talk without getting breathless. This combination gives the body time to recover, reduces strain whilst still promoting a more efficient metabolism. And you'll probably enjoy it more too.

Muscle, my friend. You were probably wondering about muscles, weren't you? You'll definitely need more metabolically active lean muscle mass to give your body new strength, shape and definition while you continue to reveal the skinnier new you. Light resistance exercises will help. Using lighter weights will help you use whole body without risk of strain or injury Lighter weights mean more repetitions and more reps will give you the lean definition that is a sure sign of a fit and healthy body.

The real challenge is getting started, taking the first step and then committing to a programme of movement and exercise. That's why it's helpful to recognise the importance of enjoying the exercise as much as possible. Find alternatives to the dreaded treadmill. Join group classes that focus on high energy movement. Take Pilates classes every week or follow a Pilates video with an excellent teacher. The body positively thrives on new and different movements so yoga and Pilates are fantastic ways to develop a stronger, more flexible body. An active yoga class, for example, that keeps your heart rate elevated can count as a cardio session and a Pilates class that incorporates added resistance from bands or weights can count as strength training.

Finally, don't forget that it's really easy to eat back all the calories you burned off at the gym in just a few unplanned minutes of pure self-indulgence. So for permanent weight loss success, combine your workouts with our Epigenetic Diet. That's an unbeatable combination for health, fitness and total wellbeing.

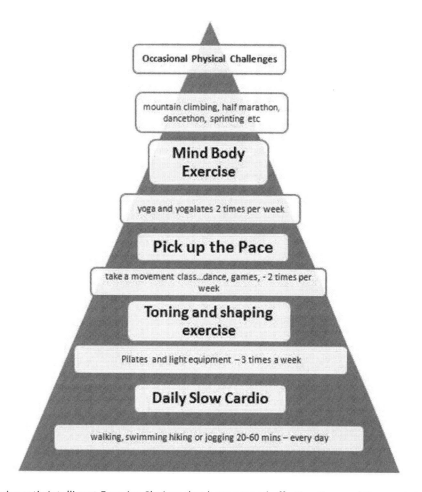

Here are the Epigenetic Intelligent Exercise Choices that have proved effective time and time again!

Walking your way to weight loss? Yes! It absolutely helps.

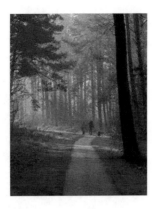

1. Walking

Walking really is an ideal exercise for weight loss even if your eyebrows just shot up in surprise! Walking really works. But it's something you have to do every single day. You don't need special equipment, you don't need special clothes, you don't even need a gym membership to do it. Just you and a pair of comfortable shoes. It's a low-impact exercise too, which reduces strain on your knees, feet and hips.

For those with obesity and heart disease, walking is an effective, low-intensity weight-loss activity that can lead to better overall health, as well as better mental wellbeing. Depending on how much you weigh, walking at a pace of four miles per hour will burn between 5 and 8 calories every minute, or between 225 and 360 calories for a 45-minute stroll. If you're interested in the maths, walking every day at this pace for 45 minutes can mean losing up to a pound a week without changing any other habits. That's every week and the accumulative effect can be truly dramatic.

So put on your walking shoes, turn up the headphones and go for a brisk stroll through the neighbourhood. If you live close to where you work or shop, make walking your primary mode of transportation and watch the excess weight slip away. Don't let the weather get in the way of your daily walk. When the weather's bad, walk indoors or take your stroll on a treadmill.

There's a lot to be said for breathing fresh air too so, if the opportunity presents itself, experience the joy of taking a walk in the woods or in the countryside. It's a good idea to take water with you too, keeping the body properly hydrated. If you aren't used to walking, take your time.

Start gently. Don't push yourself too much. Patience is a key to good exercise routines and building up your capacity to do more should leave you feeling motivated to extend your range until you can walk comfortably for as long as you wish. That in itself can mark a significant achievement and boost your confidence in your increasing levels of fitness.

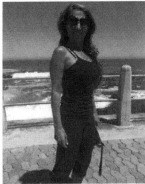

Splish splash! Come on in, the water's lovely!

2. Swimming

Swimming is such a fun way to enjoy your exercise. It's another great way to share the benefits of physical exercise and include the family as well. The great news is that this exercise works. It's really effective for weight loss and for toning. When we swim, we use all the major muscle groups, including your abdominals and back muscles, your arms, legs, hips and glutes. It's a great way of enhancing the effects of other exercises, like running and walking, or it can be your preferred form of fitness. It's also widely recognised that swimming is ideal during pregnancy, especially during the last trimester, but it's often forgotten that it's a perfect way to exercise for obese individuals and for arthritis sufferers. Water supports ninety percent of the body's weight yet provides twelve times the resistance of air so moving or swimming in the pool is a perfect way to strengthen and tone the body whilst burning calories.

Swimming has long been used as an effective tool for building stamina so you can look forward to getting fitter and building healthy reserves of energy whilst having fun in the water. Whether you're walking from side to side in the shallow end or swimming lengths, the pool is a perfect place to measure your progress. Just add an extra width or length every week and you'll be amazed how quickly your fitness levels start to climb.

Don't be square. Round is much more fun!

3. Elliptical Training

A fantastic alternative to the dreaded treadmill is the elliptical trainer, regarded by many as the better way to work out at home or at the gym. The main advantage over the conventional treadmill is that the elliptical trainer provides a low impact cardio workout that reduces strain on the key, load-bearing joints of the body. It's an ideal piece of equipment for burning calories and boosting the metabolism. Elliptical trainers have moving handles which encourage you to move your arms and give you the benefit of an upper body workout. You can select an appropriate level of resistance and intensity to match your growing levels of strength and fitness and you can expect to burn a respectable 600 calories an hour.

When you're overweight, running places enormous strain on your joints and the combination of poor posture, inadequate muscle strength and poor lumbar support is a recipe for pain and injury. The elliptical trainer is an ideal machine for allowing gentle, safe and controlled movement without stressing hips, knees and ankles. The elliptical movement that the equipment is named for reduces back strain and opens up the possibility of effective and risk free weight reduction.

As with swimming, you can increase the speed or intensity of the workout every week and build up your stamina, strength and fitness gently, carefully and effectively as the excess pounds fall away.

Not just for supermodels! Pilates really is for everyone. And that includes you!

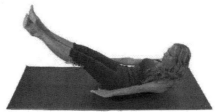

4. Pilates

As a Pilates Master Teacher and Yoga Teacher, I can vouch for the fact that Pilates especially contributes to weight loss – and so does yoga – but this indirectly as explained later on in the chapter...but look at the change in shape of my body and that is all you need to see if you are looking at getting into your best shape!

Pilates is deservedly famous for creating longer, leaner, fitter bodies. The Pilates method promotes weight loss and a leaner, more muscular appearance. But how does it work?

The precisely positioned exercise burn calories. How many calories you burn obviously depends on your body type and the level of effort.

Creating lean muscle mass, as Pilates does, is one of the best ways to increase your calorie-burning potential.

Pilates tones and shapes the whole body.

Sample some Pilates mat exercises:

One of the best ways to look and feel thinner is to have beautiful posture. Pilates creates a leaner look by emphasizing both length and better, healthier bodily alignment.

Pilates promotes deep and efficient respiration, which is essential for calorie burning and tissue regeneration.

Engaging in an exercise program, like Pilates, promotes self-esteem and heightened lifestyle consciousness. Both are associated with weight loss.

One of the most frequently asked questions about Pilates is: Will Pilates help me lose weight? The short answer is yes, Pilates is supportive but not the cause of weight loss. In many cases just beginning a Pilates class, or a home routine, is enough to jump start weight loss. However, as time goes by you may find that your body becomes accustomed to your workout level. Then, you will need to increase the intensity of your workout enough to help you continue to burn extra calories. Here are some ideas to help you ramp up your workout:

If you take a Pilates class regularly, talk to your instructor and find out if it is possible to move the class along a little more quickly. Sometimes a class needs to take that step. On the other hand, it may be that some members of your class are not ready to increase the pace of their workouts and you will have to graduate yourself to a more advanced class.

If you workout at home, it is a good idea to have a routine or two that you know quite well. That way you can focus on the breath and flow of the workout and not have to pause to review the exercise instructions or sequence.

Another great way to get a weight loss workout at home is to expand your Pilates DVD collection. Look for workouts that push your current level or add a new challenge like the magic circle, fitness band, or exercise ball. There are also a number of excellent Pilates based DVDs specifically oriented toward weight loss. As a Pilates Master Trainer I will be happy to give you a personal recommendation for good quality Pilates DVD's. Contact me at beranparry@gmail.com

Fully Commit to Each Exercise

Even if you can't move through a routine rapidly, do make sure that you get the most out of each exercise. Stretch to your fullest length at every opportunity, go for the extra scoop of the abs, breathe deeply, be precise, move with control and grace. This kind of fully engaged attitude is very much in keeping with what Joseph Pilates taught, and increases the exertion level (read weight loss potential) of your workout tremendously.

Add Equipment

Adding equipment , or different equipment, to your workout will help build muscle and strength by giving your body new challenges. Remember, muscle burns a lot of fat. If you go to a studio to workout, you could move from the mat to the reformer. If you have been using the reformer, take a chance and sign up for a class that includes a new piece of equipment, like the wunda chair or ladder barrel.

At home, smaller types of Pilates equipment such as magic circles, exercise balls and fitness bands can add the extra challenge. They also help keep your workouts interesting.

Use Less Resistance

Now here is a Pilates trick that is not used by many other fitness systems: If you are working out with Pilates resistance equipment, decrease the resistance level. This seems counter intuitive, but the instability that less resistance creates provides a significant challenge to the muscles as they attempt to maintain control and balance, especially the core muscles. This technique works very well on the reformer where you can use lighter springs, but you can apply the same principle to a lighter resistance magic circle or fitness band. You may be surprised at the level of intensity that instability can add to your workout, especially as you work to maintain precision and control during both the exertion and the release phase of an exercise, as we do in Pilates.

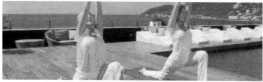

Will Doing Yoga Help Me Lose Weight?

5. Yoga

Doing yoga regularly offers many benefits, including making you feel better about your body as you become stronger and more flexible, toning your muscles, reducing stress, and improving your mental and physical well-being. But will it help you lose weight? Practicing any type of yoga will build strength, but studies show that yoga does not raise your heart rate enough to make it the only form of exercise you need to shed pounds.

In order to lose weight, you must eat correctly and burn calories by doing exercise that raises your heart rate on a regular basis. More vigorous yoga styles can provide a better workout than gentle yoga, but if weight loss is your primary goal, you will want to combine yoga with running, walking, or other aerobic exercise.

How Yoga Can Help

Yoga can still help you lose weight by bringing you to a better in tune with your body, improving your self-image and sense of well-being, and encouraging a healthy lifestyle.

If you are just starting to do yoga , are very overweight , or are quite out of shape, always choose a beginner-level class. To minimize the risk of injury, make sure find good teachers and listen to your body first and foremost.

What Kinds of Yoga Are the Most Vigorous?

The most athletic yoga styles fall in the vinyasa or flow yoga category. These styles usually start with a fast-paced series of poses called sun salutations, followed by a flow of standing poses which will keep you moving. Once you are warmed up, deeper stretches and backbends are introduced. Vinyasa includes many popular, sweaty yoga styles, such as:

Ashtanga:

Ashtanga yoga is a very vigorous style of practice and its practitioners are among the most dedicated of yogis. Beginners are often encouraged to sign up for a series of classes, which will help with motivation.

Power Yoga:

Power yoga is extremely popular at gyms and health clubs, though it is widely available at dedicated yoga studios as well. Power yoga is based on building the heat and intensity of Ashtanga while dispensing with fixed series of poses.

Hot Yoga:

Vinyasa yoga done in a hot room ups the ante by guaranteeing you'll sweat buckets. Be aware that Bikram and hot yoga are not synonymous. Bikram is a pioneering style of hot yoga, which includes a set series of poses and, indeed, a script developed by founder Bikram Choudhury. These days, there are many other styles of hot yoga that make use of the hot room but not the Bikram series.

Yoga Workouts at Home

Keep yourself exercising by doing yoga at home on the days you can't make a class. Follow along with a video if you are new to yoga. When you are ready to plan your own workouts, use these yoga sequencing ideas to help you come up with yoga sessions of varying lengths that will fit your schedule. To maximize yoga's benefits, it's great to do a little bit each day.

Your Exercise Plan and Log

Keeping an exercise log helps you stay motivated, track progress, and plan improvements. This becomes even more relevant when you have a goal like weight loss.

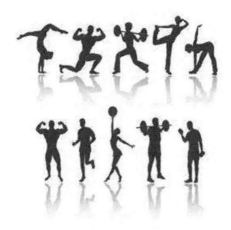

Exercise Planner and Workbook

Monday:

    am - walking 20-60 minutes or

        a slow jog or

        swimming

    pm - pilates

    eve - 10-60 minutes meditation

Tuesday:

    am - walking 20-60 minutes or

        a slow jog or

elliptical or

cycling training or

take a fun dance or movement class

pm - yoga

eve - 10-60 minutes meditation

Wednesday:

am - walking 20-60 minutes or

a slow jog or

swimming

pm - pilates

eve - 10-60 minutes meditation

Thursday:

am - walking 20-60 minutes or

a slow jog or

elliptical or

cycling training or

take a fun dance or movement class

pm - yoga

eve - 10-60 minutes meditation

Friday:

am - walking 20-60 minutes or

a slow jog or

swimming

pm - pilates

eve - 10-60 minutes meditation

Saturday:

am - walking 20-60 minutes or

a slow jog or

elliptical or

cycling training or

take a fun dance or movement class

pm -

eve - 10-60 minutes meditation

Sunday:

am - walking 20-60 minutes or

   a slow jog or

pm -

eve - 10-60 minutes meditation

Workout More Frequently

Working out more often is an obvious choice for weight loss and it can work like a charm. After all, the more opportunity you take to increase your respiration, build strength, and tone your muscles, the more weight you can lose and the trimmer you will appear

Exercise Summary

Check out a selection of exercises that are best for weight loss

The smart way to exercise is best

Walking your way to health – a fabulous daily habit!

Swimming as a safe alternative – or choose something unusual

Use Pilates to shape your body!

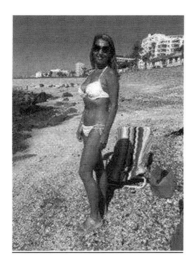

Chapter 10

Your ANTI INFLAMMATORY Epigenetic Weight Loss helpers!....Vitamin D and Magnesium

Now that you've taken the most important steps possible to take total control of your weight and give your body the best possible opportunity to feel simply amazing, it's time to introduce you to a select group of helpers that can make your programme even more effective. We're going to start with Vitamin D, the famous sunshine vitamin. Now, as you might have guessed by now, we love sharing the results of cutting edge medical and scientific research. So when we looked at the conclusions of over 3,000 independent clinical studies that have been carried out all over the world in the last year alone, we were not surprised to learn that good old Vitamin D has now been recognised as the superstar in the weight loss supplement industry.

1. Vitamin D and Weight Loss

Vitamin D is produced by the body when it's exposed to sunlight. It's a naturally occurring substance and it can also be acquired through diet or supplements. The great news is that it increases the metabolic energy of fat cells which encourages faster weight loss. Surprised? Happy to have another potent asset to help you move those excess pounds and keep you trimmer, fitter and healthier? Not only does it speed up metabolic rates for fat cells but it helps to eliminate toxins too. Now that's another great reason to ensure healthy levels of Vitamin D in your body.

FIGHTING FIBROMYALGIA With THE ANTI- INFLAMMATORY DIET By Mercedes Del Rey

One surprising insight that has emerged from the research is that both muscle and fat may well act in a similar way when it comes to storing vitamin D for future use.

New research using mathematical models has shown that a heavily muscled man and an obese man who weigh exactly the same would need the same amount of vitamin D. The key to determining how much vitamin D is appropriate for an individual would seem to be connected to body weight rather than body fat. The research is fresh so this important revelation has not been widely appreciated by most experts.

If you're overweight you're more likely to need more vitamin D than a thinner person. This new rule also applies to people with higher body weights even when it's a result of muscle mass.

Your best source for this vitamin is daily exposure to the sun, without sunblock on your skin, until your skin turns the lightest shade of pink. Too much sun is as bad as too little so don't be tempted to overdose on anything and that includes sunshine. Getting healthy exposure to the sun isn't always possible due to seasonal changes and the simple fact of where you live but moderate exposure is the ideal to aim for as it will optimize your vitamin D levels naturally.

To use the sun to maximize your vitamin D production and minimize your risk of skin damage, the middle of the day (roughly between 10:00 a.m. and 2:00 p.m.) is the best and safest time. During this UVB-intense period you will need the shortest sun exposure time to produce the most vitamin D.

If getting out into the sunshine isn't possible, you might consider using one of the safer tanning beds. These use electronic rather than magnetic ballasts and this avoids unnecessary EMF exposure. Safe tanning beds produce less of the dangerous UVA than sunlight, while unsafe ones have more UVA than sunlight. If neither of these options are available to you, then you should take an oral vitamin D3 supplement and this is where the dosage becomes important.

What's the Correct Dose of Vitamin D?

Even if you do not monitor your vitamin D levels on a regular basis, there is very little risk of taking too much. There is evidence that the safety of vitamin D is dependent on vitamin K, and that vitamin D toxicity (although very rare with the D3 form) is actually aggravated by vitamin K2 deficiency. So if you take oral vitamin D, ideally you should take vitamin K2 as well or use organic fermented foods that are high in vitamin K2, as you need about 150 mcg per day.

It must be said that it is challenging to work out precisely how much vitamin D your body produces naturally and then calculate how much you might need in supplement form. Most people are deficient in Vitamin D and the best way to correct this imbalance is to consult your doctor, take the 25 OH D blood test and then either increase your exposure to sunlight or request supplements with a dose somewhere in the range of 5,000-40,000 IU. Follow up tests should be done to check your new Vitamin D levels after a few months of taking the recommended supplements.

The latest clinical data concerning the benefits of healthy Vitamin D levels reveal that this essential chemical does a lot more than help with weight issues. It's got an impressive list of advantages for everyone:

- targets belly fat first
- turns body into fat burning mode instead of fat storing mode
- lowers high blood pressure
- helps form stronger bones to fight osteoporosis
- helps protect against different cancers
- boosts natural immune system
- reduces inflammation & joint stiffness
- influences the important hormone leptin

Calcium and the Link to Vitamin D

As you can see from the list above, there are many health benefits associated with having sufficient Vitamin D in the body. When the body experiences a lack of calcium, it is usually due to a vitamin D deficiency. This triggers the body to increase its production of synthase, a fatty acid enzyme that turns calories into fat. A calcium deficiency will cause the body to increase its synthase production by up to 500%, which may explain a further cause of obesity. When vitamin D supplements are combined with sunlight, calcium, and a low-calorie diet, it helps the body to regulate blood sugar levels, digest food properly and, for those who are interested in losing the excess pounds, it also promotes weight loss.

Recommended Intake of Vitamin D

The recommended daily intake of vitamin D should be between 400 and 600 IU. However, current research has suggested that a higher dosage would be more therapeutic. In order to improve health and heal the body, the body needs approximately 4,000 and 10,000 IU of vitamin D per day. Depending on skin tone, the body will need 10 to 20 minutes of sun every day to produce 10,000 IU of vitamin D. When the sun is not a viable option, it is best to supplement your diet with a vitamin D supplement.

2. Magnesium and Weight Loss

Obesity. Is it really connected to your epigenetic behaviour?

The popular view in the media has constantly repeated the myth that obesity is somehow inherited. People have looked at their obese relatives, sighed sadly over their bulging stomachs and resigned themselves to the apparent injustice of their bad genes. But it just isn't that simple. Oh, no. If you take a mouse with an obesity gene and deprive it of B vitamins, the obesity will be expressed. The mouse gets chubby. But if it receives plenty of B vitamins, the obese gene stays in neutral and our little mouse stays thin. The process of metabolising B vitamins is called methylation and magnesium is one of the most important elements in this process.

Magnesium plays a crucial role in many aspects of the body's health but here are some of the most relevant examples

1. Magnesium helps the body to digest, absorb, and process proteins, fats, and carbohydrates.

2. Magnesium is an essential chemical to allow insulin to open cell membranes for glucose.

3. Magnesium helps prevent obesity genes from expressing themselves.

Magnesium and THE WEIGHT CONNECTION

Magnesium and the B-complex vitamins are important for helping to access the energy that's contained within our food. They're responsible for switching on enzymes that control digestion, nutrient absorption and the way we process proteins, fats, and carbohydrates. When our bodies don't get enough of these essential nutrients, we can experience a surprising range of negative consequences. Some of the unexpected consequences include hypoglycaemia, anxiety, depression and even our old friend, obesity.

The fact is that amidst an extraordinary array of foods and an incredible choice of what and how much to eat, we are often starved of essential nutrients. There is a fascinating research project that has identified the connection between our food cravings for foods and the way our bodies lack those essential nutrients.

Processed foods that lack the essential nutritional content that supports healthy metabolism are effectively empty calories. They only serve to add unhealthy weight to the body without contributing to the body's total nutritional requirements. So, as a result, you're often really hungry. So you keep eating. But you're still hungry and your body's packing on the extra weight but in reality you're starved of good nutrition.

The study suggested that changing to a healthy diet can re-set the brain's triggers for high fat, high calorie food and create a much healthier response to food choices that avoids over-eating and focuses on a naturally low-fat, high energy diet. You just know that's going to help to keep the unwanted weight off and introduce you to a whole new world of feeling great.

Magnesium also produces the metabolic reaction that instructs insulin to allow the transfer of energy-providing glucose into our cells. If the body doesn't have enough magnesium to fulfil this important role, both insulin and glucose levels increase. The excess glucose is converted into fat and this obviously contributes to obesity problems. Having excess insulin also raises the risk of diabetes.

Is stress connected to weight gain? Oh yes it is. But we have the answer!

The powerful connection between stress and obesity has long been understood. When our bodies are stressed, we produce more of the chemical cortisol and the cortisol effectively forces a metabolic reversal that makes weight loss almost impossible. The great news is that our good friend and helper, magnesium, can effectively neutralise these undesirable effects of stress.

ABDOMINAL Fat - Is a corset the only answer? No!!

Gaining weight around your middle is strongly related to magnesium deficiency and an inability to properly utilise insulin. This is when we run the risk of encountering Syndrome X. You only need a tape measure to diagnose a predisposition to Syndrome X. If you have a waist size above 40 inches in men and above 35 in women then you're at risk. In their book The Magnesium Factor, authors Mildred Seelig, M.D., and Andrea Rosanoff, Ph.D.,

FIGHTING FIBROMYALGIA With THE ANTI- INFLAMMATORY DIET By Mercedes Del Rey

refer to research that demonstrates over half the insulin in the bloodstream is directed at abdominal tissue. They suggest that as more and more insulin is produced to deal with a high-sugar diet, abdominal size increases mainly to process the extra insulin.

Magnesium and SYNDROME X

The term "syndrome X" refers to a set of conditions that are really the product of long-standing nutritional deficiency, especially magnesium deficiency. Syndrome X is simply the result of starving the body of those essential nutrients. The long list of problems includes high cholesterol, hypertension and obesity. It also includes elevated triglyccrides and high levels of uric acid. High triglycerides are usually found when cholesterol levels are too high but it happens most often with people who consume a daily high-sugar diet and that includes fizzy drinks, cakes, biscuits, candy and pastries. Syndrome X is a description of what happens when we eat badly.

Vitamins and minerals are the driving forces that produce our metabolism. Without them, we get problems. So, the first step in treating non-specific symptoms is to consider diet and dietary supplements, not drugs. It is also important to note that many of the diets that people adopt to lose weight are often deficient in the vital ingredient that can make such an important contribution to weight control - magnesium.

We mentioned above that magnesium is an essential part of the process that allows insulin to play its part in the way that glucose is transferred into our cells. The cells need that energy to function normally so, if there isn't enough magnesium, the cells can't absorb the glucose and this is what follows:

1. Glucose levels become elevated.
2. Glucose is stored as fat and leads to obesity.
3. Elevated glucose leads to diabetes.
4. Obesity puts a strain on the heart.
5. Excess glucose becomes attached to certain proteins (glycated), leading to kidney damage, neuropathy, blindness, and other diabetic complications.
6. Insulin-resistant cells don't allow magnesium into the cells.
7. Further magnesium deficiency leads to hypertension.
8. Magnesium deficiency leads to cholesterol build-up and both these conditions are implicated in heart disease.

Syndrome X, according to Dr. Gerald Reaven, the individual who coined the term, may be responsible for a large percentage of the heart and artery disease that occurs today. Unquestionably, magnesium deficiency is a major factor in the origins of each of its signs and symptoms, from elevated triglycerides and obesity to disturbed insulin metabolism.

INSULIN RESISTANCE

FIGHTING FIBROMYALGIA With THE ANTI- INFLAMMATORY DIET By Mercedes Del Rey

Food. Food. Glorious Food.

We've made lots of references and observations about food. Well, it's one of the keys to truly great weight management. It's time now to take a closer look at the way that specific foods can make you gain unwanted weight at an alarming rate and stack the fat around your belly.

Insulin is a very powerful hormone and, as you might expect, it can produce very powerful reactions in humans. You've probably seen news items and articles referring to the glycemic index. Foods that feature at the top of this index are a cause of massive increases in insulin secretion and this produces intense cravings, hunger and an increase in fat production. Foods that score high on the glycemic index are a disaster for healthy weight control and a menace to good health. There's a great deal of debate about saturated or unsaturated fats. All of these components have some level of importance. However, nutritionists and doctors virtually never mention the most important and significant components of food which can lead to weight gain and obesity. We need to lift the lid right now on food processing techniques

We've identified a key role that insulin plays in the body: it opens up sites on cell membranes to allow the flow of glucose, a cell's source of energy. Cells that no longer respond to the signals from insulin and refuse the entry of glucose are called insulin-resistant. As a result, blood glucose levels rise and the body produces more and more insulin. Glucose and insulin are pumped around the body, causing tissue damage that results in further depletion of magnesium, an increased risk of heart disease and the likelihood of adult onset diabetes.

So, get your weight loss cure today. Start taking magnesium, soak in Epsom Bath Salts or spray it on your body and watch the weight drop off. Sometimes it really is the simplest things that can make the most dramatic difference. In this case, we're highlighting magnesium as one of the best allies we can recruit to our weight control cause.

Helpers - Summary

1. The power of sunshine and the Vitamin D connection
2. Magnesium and weight loss
3. Syndrome X
4. Insulin resistance
5. Relieving health issues with smart nutrition

Disclaimer:

The information you have read in this chapter needs to be matched with your current medical status to determine how to use these fantastic weight loss aids safely and effectively. Please consult with a Functional Medicine Specialist in order to take these supplements safely. I will be happy to recommend a suitable professional in your area. Just contact me on beranparry@gmail.com

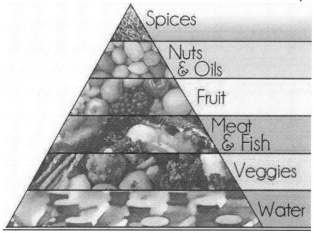

Chapter 11

Paleo – Keto -Epigenetic ANTI INFLAMMATORY DELICIOUS DAILY FOOD AND DINING OUT GUIDE

Your Personal Guide to a Leaner New You is full of the latest research on how your body really works. We've armed and prepared you with the science, the knowledge and the facts about intelligent, effective weight control and now we want to expand your knowledge further by sharing a great list of things that you can eat and enjoy plus a list of the unhelpful things that you really cannot afford to have in your diet if you plan to control your weight and discover the real meaning of total health. You're going to be a great detective and find all the clues to what you're really eating by reading the labels on your food.

Sugar, my little sweetie, is always off the menu. Just because the amount listed is very small, it's still sugar and you have to look for every form of sweetener, real or artificial, because if it's on the label it just isn't going into your mouth. Sugar is out. Gone. Adios, amigo. Forever.

Almond Flour. "You can make flour from almonds?" Yes you can and you can eat it. People are discovering the benefits of coconut flour too because these flours do not come from grains. That makes them much safer alternatives to the traditional flour that contains inflammatory-provoking glutens. It's even possible to make almond milk too but the commercially produced variety usually contains sweeteners so gets disqualified before you even open the carton. If in doubt, it's better to make your own almond milk and that way you can absolutely control the purity of the ingredients. The controversial use of almond flour is to use it as a substitute for baking bread, biscuits or anything else where we would previously have used regular flour. In cleansing the body, it might not be appropriate to use almond or coconut flour for baking. Sorry.

Bacon is incredibly popular because it tastes so good. One of the reasons for that great flavour is that the meat processors often add sugar as a preservative and flavour enhancer. Sourcing hormone-free and antibiotic-free meat is a real challenge so bacon is definitely off the menu.

Bean sprouts have been a staple of the vegetarian diet since records began but it's the plant that is good to eat, not the seeds. The beans contain compounds that are difficult for humans to digest successfully. So it's a resounding yes to the sprouts and no to the beans themselves.

Bread. You're not serious, are you? Did you expect a green light for bread? Sorry, folks. It's definitely a no. Make that a capital N-O just to be certain. If you miss the old demon slice of toxicity, try using almond flour, sweet potato flour or flaxseed flour as your new basic ingredient for making a dramatically healthier alternative to grain-based bread.

Buckwheat might surprise you because it's long been associated with the image of a healthy diet. Buckwheat though is a pseudo cereal. Technically speaking, it isn't a grain but it still causes similar problems to all the grains we're eliminating from our daily diet. So buckwheat goes onto the No pile.

Cocoa. At last we've found something tasty that we can consume! Pure cocoa is fine as long as - you guessed it! - it does not contain any sugar or sweeteners. It's increasingly being used as a flavour enhancer with people adding it to their coffee and tea and even incorporating it in spices and sauces to accompany meat dishes. More versatile than you might imagine and a welcome guest on the menu!

Carob. Often used as a substitute for chocolate, this legume is usually consumed as carob powder. Happily the powder is made from the pod rather than the potentially harmful seed of the carob. So as long as you avoid the seeds, carob is a good food choice as far as healthy eating is concerned.

Chia. These are another great choice is a healthy eating plan. Chia seeds are not part of the same family of seeds that we find in grains and legumes so they're fine to eat.

Citric Acid. We often find it used as a preservative in canned produce and in jars of preserved foods. Amongst all the harmful substances that are used as food additives, citric acid stands out as one of the few products that is completely acceptable.

Coconut water. It's naturally sweet and delicious but you must check the label to make absolutely sure there is no added sugar. It is not a substitute for fizzy drinks so it's important to limit your consumption. And it isn't a replacement for your daily quota of water. But it is on the goodie list so it's OK to drink and enjoy.

Coffee is good for you. Pure, organic coffee is a potent anti-oxidant and has been linked to a variety of health benefits. Just make sure you don't add sugar, sweeteners, artificial flavourings or milk.

Chocolate is an addictive substance and is the drug of choice for many people. But if you opt for the sugar-free, dairy-free, dark varieties with at least 70% cocoa, you can enjoy your addiction - always in moderation! - with a clear conscience.

Dates contain high quantities of naturally occurring sugar so Keto says NO!

Flax seeds are not part of the same group of seeds that are linked to grains, which means that they are a fine source of nutrition.

French fries are a particularly unhealthy way to enjoy potatoes. The problem lies in the fact that they are fried in vegetable oil and this is off limits to anyone seeking to control their weight and boost their wellbeing. If you make your own fries at home, you can use coconut oil instead of vegetable oil or you can bake them or roast them to avoid the frying problem altogether.

Fruit juice is off the agenda. That's right. Fruit juice delivers way too much sugar to your bloodstream way too quickly and produces a massive insulin reaction. Not good! The only way to enjoy fruit juice is when it's still inside the fruit. The body has to work a lot harder to extract the energy from the fruit pulp and this slows down the absorption rate of the sugars, avoiding the sudden sugar rush and the subsequent dramatic fall off as the insulin kicks in. There's an enormous amount of advertising surrounding the supposed health benefits of drinking fruit juice. It's giving you the wrong information. Stick to the fruit instead and live longer.

Guar gum is a natural thickener and it's a perfectly acceptable item on your food list.

Green beans get our yes vote despite the fact that they're a legume and contain seeds. But green beans have very small, immature seeds inside a large green pod so the potential for damage is correspondingly small.

Hemp seeds are a great source of healthy protein. They're not related to the harmful seeds that occur in grains so you're free to add hemp seeds to your diet plan and enjoy the benefits.

Hummus always looks so healthy but it's made from a not so healthy legume, the garbanzo bean or chick pea. It seems tough, but hummus just got fired from the list.

Mayonnaise usually contains sugar. I know. It's everywhere. Even the healthy-sounding olive oil based mayo is largely made up from soybean oil so your best alternative is to make your own. It really is fast and easy. Organic eggs (one yolk) and extra virgin olive oil (one cup), a little apple cider vinegar(2 teaspoons), a pinch of garlic powder and black pepper to taste...and you'll be amazed how great real mayo tastes.

Mustard is a great gift to many meals, adding some much-needed flavour to otherwise bland and tasteless dishes. Just be careful about the label. Some manufacturers add flavourings, sugar, colouring agents and wine. Pure and natural are your watchwords. Once again make your own with a seed grinder, one cup ground (semi) mustard seeds, two tablespoons olive oil, one tablespoon apple cider vinegar and stevia to taste.

Potatoes are a surprising candidate for healthy eating. IN MODERATION. You can eat them, of course, but you are much better off with the small red skinned potatoes and you need to eat them sparingly. Needless to say perhaps, but you need to avoid the commercially prepared, deep fried potato chips or French fries.

Protein shakes have become increasingly popular as the protein diet fashion has persuaded countless individuals to use a scoop of protein powder as a substitute for intelligent nutrition. But have you read the ingredients on the label? Protein shakes are full of the things you really need to avoid if you're planning on losing weight and getting seriously healthy. The only exception to the rule is our old friend hemp. Hemp protein powder can be a useful assistant in your health and wellbeing plan because your body works so well with this potent little seed.

Quinoa can be found filling the shelves in health stores everywhere but it can act very much like a grain and produce similarly harmful effects. Quinoa just got cancelled. The same applies to buckwheat, amaranth and other gluten-free grain substitutes.

Safflower or sunflower oil is also off the menu because we want to cut out vegetable oils as much as possible.

Salt is an important part of the human diet. You might not know that iodised table salt also contains a sugar in the form of dextrose. This sugar is used to block the oxidisation process that would effectively neutralise the potassium iodine that's an important part of iodised salt. You still need salt in your diet and it's almost impossible to eat outside of the house without encountering iodised salt: it's added to restaurant and processed food as standard.

Smoothies get top marks for health as long as they're based on fresh vegetables, health coconut milk or almond milk but... no colourants, unnatural flavourings or artificial additives.

Stevia is the only sweetener that passes our healthy additive test. It's natural and we recommend the less-processed leaf rather than the alcohol based liquid or powder versions. Stevia Glycerite which is alcohol free is the best I have used.

Tahini is made from sesame seeds and gets a welcome 'Yes' on our list of acceptable, healthy foods. Plus it tastes really, really great!

Vanilla extract is such a favourite flavour enhancer in so many baking recipes but it usually contains sugar or alcohol. The extract is a no-no but you can use vanilla bean powder to get the super flavour without the sugar or alcohol additives.

PKE DINING GUIDE

Whether by choice or profession, you will at some point find yourself at a restaurant, with the challenge of what to eat. Restaurant menus can be a confusing territory – but these tips will make your healthy dining experience fun, satisfying, and stress-free.

Ahead of time

- Call ahead to make sure the restaurant will cope with your requirements.
- When dining with a group, take charge and suggest a restaurant that meets your specifications.
- Smaller, local restaurants are generally more accommodating to substitutions or customization than larger chains.
- Research the menu beforehand and plan your order so you won't be tempted by other less healthy dishes when you arrive.
- Pack your own small bottle of dressing. Don't make a big deal out of it and most servers won't say anything.

When seated

- Upon being seated, ask the server not to serve you bread.
- Don't hesitate to ask about food sourcing, hidden ingredients (like cheese on a salad), or preparation methods.
- Be specific about any allergies, sensitivities, or preferences, especially if you experience health consequences when exposed – write them down for the chef if there is confusion.

Ordering

- Be firm but nice about your requests. Say things like, "Would it be possible…?" or "I'd love it if…"
- Get creative! Order sandwiches without bread, pasta toppings on a bed of spinach, or double vegetables as your side.
- If you've got wild-caught or organic protein options, choose those above conventionally raised protein.
- Ask for vegetables to be steamed or sautéed with olive oil, instead of cooked or fried in vegetable oil.
- Omelets are often infused with milk or pancake batter (!) to make them fluffier. Request boiled eggs, or order them poached.
- Request individual bottles of olive oil and vinegar and some fresh lemon to use as a dressing on salad, vegetables, or protein.

Bill, please

- When you have a good experience, thank the server and the chef – and tip well, especially if the restaurant is one you visit often.
- Relax about being assertive with your demands – you are the customer after all!
- Make it a top priority to never be compromised in a restaurant again!

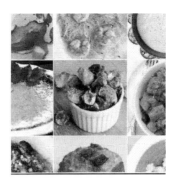

Chapter 12

Index to ANTI INFLAMMATORY Recipes

BREAKFASTS – No Grain

1. Gutsy Granola

2. High Protein Breakfast Gold

3. Divine Protein Muesli

4. Ultimate Skinny Granola

5. Sweetie Skinny Crackers

EGGIE MEALS

1. Scrambled Eggs with Chilli

2. Spicy Scrambled Eggs

3. Spicy India Omelet

4. Spectacular Spinach Omelet

5. Outstanding Veggie Omelette

MAIN COURSE - CHICKEN

1. Spicy Turkey Stir Fry

2. Roasted Lemon Herb Chicken

3. Basil Turkey with Roasted Tomatoes

4. Sexy Turkey Scramble

5. Sensational Courgette Pasta and Turkey Bolognese

MAIN COURSE – FISH

1. Divine Prawn Mexicana

2. Superior Salmon with Lemon and Thyme OR Use any White fish

3. Spectacular Shrimp Scampi in Spaghetti Sauce

4. Scrumptious Cod in Delish Sauce

5. Mouthwatering Stuffed Salmon

SALAD – ANIMAL PROTEIN

1. Rosy Chicken Supreme Salad

2. Sexy Italian Tuna Salad

3. Skinny Chicken salad

4. Turkey Taco Salad

5. Cheeky Turkey Salad

PURE VEGETABLES – PLEASE ADD ANY RAW NUTS and/or AVOCADO TO OBTAIN THE KETO FAT REQUIREMENT ON ALL THESE RECIPES!

1. Rucola Salad

2. Tasty Spring Salad

3. Pure Delish Spinach Salad

4. Sexy Salsa Salad

5. Jalapeno Salsa

DESERTS

1. Fabulous Brownie Treats

2. Pristine Pumpkin Divine

3. Spectacular Spinach Brownies

4. Chestnut- Cacao Cake

5. Choco Cookie Delight

SMOOTHIES

1. Voluptuous Vanilla Hot Drink

2. Almond Butter Smoothies

3. Baby Kale Pineapple Smoothie

4. Vanilla Blueberry Smoothie

5. Zesty Citrus Smoothie

SNACKS

1. Delectable Parsnip Chips

2. Skinny Power Snack

3. Gummy Citrus Snack

4. Gorgeous Spicy Nuts

5. Spicy Pumpkin Seed Bonanza

SOUPS

1. Cheeky Chicken Soup

2. Ginger Carrot Delight Soup

3. Wonderful Watercress Soup

4. Celery Cashew Cream Soup

5. Mighty Andalusian Gazpacho

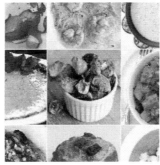

Chapter 13

The ANTI INFLAMMATORY 3 WEEK Plan

How the PKE Weight Loss Plan Works: The Basics

The Plan is a 3 week life changing eating program, meaning that you will be eating pure, healthy Paleo-Keto-Epigenetic options for a full 16 week period to achieve the maximum permanent benefits. You will not be hungry!

Mornings:

An energy-dense egg based cooked breakfast, or an SDD smoothie and/or an SDD non grain muesli option

Lunches:

A light but filling salad or paleo meal concentrating on your anti-oxidants salads, green leafy vegetables …..An epigenetic protein selection is included in the salad.

Dinners:

A hearty protein based cooked meal or a filling protein soup twice a week

Lunch and Dinner Swops:

Always possible!

Treats & Snacks:

See our extensive recipe section for a selection of high-performance healthy snacks that you can make at home! Also, any combination of low sugar fruits, berries, nuts and seeds are great to include.

Hydration:

Remember to keep yourself fully hydrated by consuming between 6-8 cups of fresh water throughout the day. You can also supplement this diet by including additional smoothies

IMPORTANT: On Protein Soup Evenings make sure you eat your second daily snack in the afternoon and then ensure you have no solid food after your protein soup until the next morning.

Week 1

DAY 1
Breakfast
    Gutsy Granola
Lunch
    Spicy Turkey Stir Fry
Snacks
    Delectable Parsnip Chips
Dinner
    Divine Prawn Mexicana
Dessert
    Fabulous Brownie Treats

DAY 2
Breakfast
    Baby Kale Pineapple Smoothie
Lunch
    Sexy Italian Tuna Salad
Snacks
    Spicy Pumpkin Seed Bonanza
Dinner
    Roasted Lemon Herb Chicken
Dessert
    Pristine Pumpkin Divine

DAY 3
Breakfast
    Outstanding Veggie Omelette
Lunch
    Cheeky Chicken Soup
Snacks
    Gummy Citrus Snack
Dinner
    Sensational Courgette Pasta and Turkey Bolognaise

Dessert

Choco Cookie Delight

DAY 4

Breakfast

High Protein Breakfast Gold

Lunch

Skinny Chicken Salad

Snacks

Skinny Power Snacks

Dinner

Spicy Turkey Stir Fry

Dessert

Chestnut Cacao Cake

DAY 5

Breakfast

Voluptuous Vanilla Hot Drink

Lunch

Divine Prawn Mexicana

Snacks

Gorgeous Spicy Nuts

Dinner

Sexy Turkey Scramble

Dessert

Spectacular Spinach Brownies

DAY 6

Breakfast

Spicy India Omelette

Lunch

Turkey Taco Salad

Snacks

Spicy Pumpkin Seed Bonanza

Dinner

Mighty Andalusian Gazpacho

Dessert

Choco Cookie Delight

DAY 7

Breakfast

Divine Protein Muesli

Lunch

Scrumptious Cod in Delish Sauce

Snacks

Spicy Pumpkin Seed Bonanza

Dinner

Mouth-watering Stuffed Salmon

Dessert

Fabulous Brownie Treats

WEEK 2

DAY 1
Breakfast
      Zesty Citrus Smoothie
Lunch
      Rosy Chicken Supreme Salad
Snacks
      Delectable Parsnip Chips
Dinner
      Basil Turkey with Roasted Tomatoes
Dessert
      Pristine Pumpkin Divine

DAY 2
Breakfast
      Outstanding Veggie Omelette
Lunch
      Superior Salmon with Lemon and Thyme OR Use any White fish
Snacks
      Skinny Power Snack
Dinner
      Sensational Courgette Pasta and Turkey Bolognaise
Dessert
      Choco Cookie Delight

DAY 3
Breakfast
      Gutsy Granola
Lunch
      Spicy Turkey Stir Fry
Snacks
      Skinny Power Snacks
Dinner
      Spectacular Shrimp Scampi in Spaghetti Sauce
Dessert
      Chestnut- Cacao Cake

DAY 4
Breakfast
      Vanilla Blueberry Smoothie
Lunch
      Cheeky Chicken Soup
Snacks
      Gorgeous Spicy Nuts

FIGHTING FIBROMYALGIA With THE ANTI- INFLAMMATORY DIET By Mercedes Del Rey

Dinner
Superior Salmon with Lemon and Thyme OR Use any White fish
Dessert
Choco Cookie Delight

DAY 5
Breakfast
Spicy Scrambled Eggs
Lunch
Turkey Taco Salad
Snacks
Gummy Citrus Snack
Dinner
Roasted Lemon Herb Chicken
Dessert
Spectacular Spinach Brownies

DAY 6
Breakfast
Ultimate Skinny Granola
Lunch
Sexy Turkey Scramble
Snacks
Jalapeno Salsa
Dinner
Divine Prawn Mexicana
Dessert
Chestnut- Cacao Cake

DAY 7
Breakfast
Almond Butter Smoothies
Lunch
Basil Turkey with Roasted Tomatoes
Snacks
Pure Delish Spinach Salad
Dinner
Spectacular Shrimp Scampi in Spaghetti Sauce
Dessert
Spectacular Spinach Brownies

FIGHTING FIBROMYALGIA With THE ANTI- INFLAMMATORY DIET By Mercedes Del Rey
WEEK 3

DAY 1
Breakfast
Spectacular Spinach Omelet
Lunch
Sexy Salsa Salad
Snacks
Skinny Power Snack
Dinner
Mouth-watering Stuffed Salmon
Dessert
Pristine Pumpkin Divine

DAY 2
Breakfast
Divine Protein Muesli
Lunch
Sexy Italian Tuna Salad
Snacks
Gorgeous Spicy Nuts
Dinner
Roasted Lemon Herb Chicken
Dessert
Spectacular Spinach Brownies

DAY 3
Breakfast
Vanilla Blueberry Smoothie
Lunch
Basil Turkey with Roasted Tomatoes
Snacks
Tasty Spring Salad
Dinner
Sensational Courgette Pasta and Turkey Bolognaise
Dessert
Choco Cookie Delight

DAY 4
Breakfast
Outstanding Veggie Omelette
Lunch
Divine Prawn Mexicana
Snacks
Skinny Power Snack

127

Dinner
        Sexy Turkey Scramble
Dessert
        Fabulous Brownie Treats

DAY 5
Breakfast
        Sweetie Skinny Crackers
Lunch
        Cheeky Chicken Soup
Snacks
        Pure Delish Spinach Salad
Dinner
        Roasted Lemon Herb Chicken
Dessert
        Pristine Pumpkin Divine

DAY 6
Breakfast
        Baby Kale Pineapple Smoothie
Lunch
        Rosy Chicken Supreme Salad
Snacks
        Spicy Pumpkin Seed Bonanza
Dinner
        Sensational Courgette Pasta and Turkey Bolognaise
Dessert
        Chestnut- Cacao Cake

DAY 7
Breakfast
        Spectacular Spinach Omelette
Lunch
        Skinny Chicken Salad
Snacks
        Delectable Parsnip Chips
Dinner
        Superior Salmon with Lemon and Thyme – OR - Use any White fish
Dessert
        Choco Cookie Delight

Chapter 14

ANTI INFLAMMATORY RECIPES

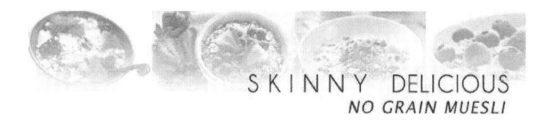

ANTI INFLAMMATORY Breakfasts (Grain Free)

1. Gutsy Granola

Ingredients:
1 cup cashews
3/4 cup almonds
1/4 cup pumpkin seeds, shelled
1/4 cup sunflower seeds, shelled
1/2 cup unsweetened coconut flakes
1/4 cup coconut oil
Stevia to taste
1 tsp vanilla
low sodium salt to taste

Instructions:
Preheat oven to 300 degrees F. Line a baking sheet with parchment paper. Place the cashews, almonds, coconut flakes and pumpkin seeds into a blender and pulse to break the mixture into smaller pieces.

In a large microwave-safe bowl, melt the coconut oil, vanilla, and stevia together for 40-50 seconds. Add in the mixture from the blender and the sunflower seeds, and stir to coat.

Spread the mixture out onto the baking sheet and cook for 20-25 minutes, stirring once, until the mixture is lightly browned. Remove from heat. Add low sodium salt.

Press the granola mixture together to form a flat, even surface.

Cool for about 15 minutes, and then break into pieces.

2. High Protein Breakfast Gold

Ingredients:
1/2 cup (c). Flax-Meal, golden
1/2 c. Chia seed
Stevia liquid to taste
2 tbs. dark ground cinnamon
1 tbs. hemp protein powder
2 tbs. coconut oil, melted
1 tsp. vanilla extract
3/4 c. + 2 tbs. hot water

Instructions:
Begin to spread the dough out until its super thin, onto a parchment paper lined cookie sheet. Bake at 325 for 15 minutes, then drop it down to 300 and leave for 30 minutes.

Before dropping it, pull out the sheet and cut it. Put it back into the oven exactly like this, don't separate the pieces.

When the 30 minutes are up, pull it out and separate the pieces.

Drop the pieces to 200 degrees F for 1 hour. They will be completely dried out at this point.

Enjoy with almond or other nut milk!

3. Divine Protein Muesli

Ingredients:
1 cup unsweetened unsulfured coconut flakes
1 tbsp chopped walnuts
1 tbsp raw almonds (~10)
1 tbsp chocolate chips (dark and sugar free)
1/2 tsp cinnamon
1 cup unsweetened almond milk
1 scoop hemp protein

Instructions:
In a medium bowl layer coconut flakes, walnuts, almonds and chocolate chips.

Sprinkle with cinnamon.

Pour cold almond milk over the muesli and eat with a spoon.

4. Ultimate Skinny Granola

Ingredients:
1 cup of unsweetened coconut milk or unsweetened almond milk
Stevia liquid to taste
1 tablespooneach of unsalted …
pecan pieces
walnut pieces
almonds
pistachios
raw pine nuts
raw sunflower/safflower seeds
raw pumpkin seeds
2 Tablespoons of frozen or fresh berry selection (e.g. blueberries, blackberries, raspberries, strawberries, or other kinds etc)

Instructions:
Put all the nuts & seeds in a breakfast bowl.

add a few drops of pure liquid stevia and stir it well in.

Add the berries and milk.

If using frozen berries, wait for 2-3 minutes for them to get warmer.

The berries will now release some color into the milk, making it look really interesting.

Enjoy!

5. Sweetie Skinny Crackers

Ingredients:
1 egg
pure liquid stevia to taste
1 Tbspn coconut oil, melted
1.5 cups almond flour
.5 cup coconut flour
1 teaspoon cinnamon

Instructions:
Preheat oven to 350°

In a large bowl, whisk together the egg, pure liquid stevia and melted coconut oil

Add the coconut and almond flour and stir to combine.

Give the dough a couple of kneads so it's well incorporated.

Turn the dough onto a piece of parchment paper and flatten a bit with your hands.

Place another piece of parchment on top and roll out with a rolling pin until it's about 1/8 inch thick.

Remove the top piece of parchment and cut the dough into 1/4 inch squares for cereal, and about 2"x3" for crackers

Sprinkle the cinnamon into the dough mixture.

Slide the dough with the bottom parchment paper onto a baking sheet and bake for 15 minutes.

Turn down the oven to 325° and bake for another 10-15 minutes, or until the cereal / crackers are crisp.

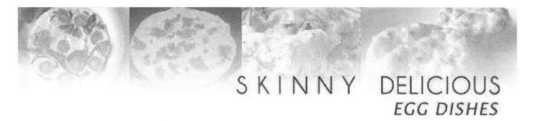

SKINNY DELICIOUS
EGG DISHES

ANTI INFLAMMATORY Egg Meals

1. Scrambled Eggs with Chilli

Ingredients:
4 fresh green chillies with skins removed
2 tablespoons (30g or 1 oz) coconut oil
1 small onion, peeled and finely chopped
6 eggs
1/4 cup (62ml or 2 fl oz) coconut milk
low sodium salt to taste

Instructions:
After removing chilli skins, remove and discard seeds and finely chop remaining chilli.

Beat eggs, coconut milk and salt in a bowl and set aside.

Heat oil in a medium size saucepan over a medium heat.

Reduce heat to low and add egg mixture to saucepan and mix well.

Scatter chilies over mixture.

Cook over a low heat until eggs are cooked.

Serves 4. Serve hot.

2. Spicy Scrambled Eggs

Ingredients:
1 tablespoon extra virgin olive oil
1 red onion, finely chopped
1 medium green pepper, cored, seeded, and finely chopped
1 chilli, seeded and cut into thin strips
3 ripe tomatoes, peeled, seeded, and chopped
Salt and freshly ground black pepper
4 large organic eggs

Instructions:
Heat the olive oil in a large, heavy, preferably nonstick skillet over medium heat.

Add the onion and cook until soft, 6 to 7 minutes.

Add the pepper and chilli and continue cooking until soft, another 4 to 5 minutes.

Add in the tomatoes, and salt and pepper to taste and cook uncovered, over low heat for 10 minutes.

Add the eggs, stirring them into the mixture to distribute.

Cover the skillet and cook until the eggs are set but still fluffy and tender, about 7 to 8 minutes. Divide between 4 plates and serve.

3. Spicy India Omelet

Ingredients:
3 Eggs
1 Onion, chopped
4 Green Chilli (optional)
1/4 cup Coconut grated
Low sodium Salt as required
1 tblspoon olive oil

Instructions:
Beat the Eggs severely.

Mix chopped onion, rounded green chilli, salt and grated coconuts with eggs.

Heat oil on a medium-low heat, in a pan.

Pour the mixture in the form of pancakes and cook it on the both sides.

4. Spectacular Spinach Omelet

Ingredients:
2 eggs
1.5 cups raw spinach
coconut oil, about 1 tbsp
1/3 c tomatoes and onion salsa (lightly fried in pan)
1 tbsp fresh cilantro

Instructions:
Melt coconut oil on medium in frying pan. Add spinach, cook until mostly wilted. Beat eggs and add to pan.

Flip once the egg sets around the edge. When it's almost done add the salsa on top just to warm it. Move to plate and add cilantro. Serves one.

5. Outstanding Veggie Omelette

Ingredients:
3 eggs, beaten
1 carrot, matchstick cut
3 scallions, diagonal sliced
1 handful tiny broccoli florets or whatever leftover veggies you have
Bits of leftover cooked turkey
Safflower oil
Low sodium salt

Instructions:
Heat oil in a wok or large cast iron skillet over medium heat, until hot enough to sizzle a drop of water.

Add broccoli and carrots, stir fry 2 min. until soft.

Add cooked turkey, stir fry 1 min. until heated through.
Add scallions and eggs, scramble.
Add salt to taste. Serve.

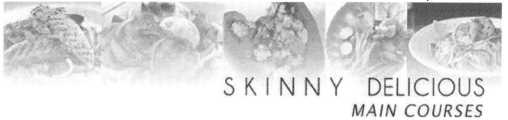

SKINNY DELICIOUS
MAIN COURSES

ANTI INFLAMMATORY Main Meals (Lunch or Dinner)

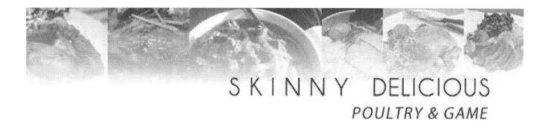

SKINNY DELICIOUS
POULTRY & GAME

ANTI INFLAMMATORY Poultry & Game

1. Spicy Turkey Stir Fry

Ingredients:
2 lbs. boneless skinless chicken or turkey breasts, cut into 1-inch slices
2 tbsp coconut oil
1 tsp cumin seeds
1/2 each green, red, and orange bell pepper, thinly sliced
1 tsp garam masala
2 tsp freshly ground pepper
low sodium salt, to taste
Scallions, for garnish

For the marinade:
1/2 cup coconut cream
1 clove garlic, minced
1 tsp ginger, minced
1 tbsp freshly ground pepper

2 tsp low sodium salt

1/4 tsp turmeric

Instructions:

Place all of the marinade ingredients into a Ziploc bag. Add the chicken, close the bag, and shake to coat.

Marinate in the refrigerator for at least 30 minutes, or up to 6 hours.

In a wok or large sauté pan, melt the coconut oil over medium-high heat.

Add the cumin seeds and cook for 2-3 minutes.

Add the marinated chicken/turkey and let cook for 5 minutes. Stir the chicken/turkey until it begins to brown, and then add the peppers, garam masala, and freshly ground pepper.

Sprinkle with low sodium salt. Cook for 4-5 minutes, stirring regularly, or until the bell pepper is cooked to desired doneness. Serve hot.

2. Roasted Lemon Herb Chicken

Ingredients:
12 total pieces bone-in chicken thighs and legs
1 medium onion, thinly sliced
1 tbsp dried rosemary
1 tsp dried thyme
1 lemon, sliced thin
1 orange, sliced thin

For the marinade:
5 tbsp extra virgin olive oil
6 cloves garlic, minced
Stevia to taste
Juice of 1 lemon
Juice of 1 orange
1 tbsp Italian seasoning – salt free
1 tsp onion powder
Dash of red pepper flakes
low sodium salt and freshly ground pepper, to taste

Instructions:
Whisk together all of the marinade ingredients in a small bowl. Place the chicken in a baking dish (or a large Ziploc bag) and pour the marinade over it. Marinate for 3 hours to overnight.

Preheat the oven to 400 degrees F. Place the chicken in a baking dish and arrange with the onion, orange, and lemon slices.

Sprinkle with thyme, rosemary, low sodium salt and pepper. Cover with aluminum foil and bake for 30 minutes.

Remove the foil, baste the chicken, and bake for another 30 minutes uncovered, until the chicken is cooked through.

3. Basil Turkey with Roasted Tomatoes

Ingredients:
2 turkey breasts
1 cup mushrooms, chopped
1/2 medium onion, chopped
1-2 tbsp extra virgin olive oil
Half cup thinly sliced fresh basil
low sodium salt and pepper, to taste
1 pint cherry tomatoes
Stevia to taste
Fresh parsley, for garnish

Instructions:
Preheat the oven to 400 degrees F.

Place the tomatoes on a baking sheet and drizzle with olive oil and stevia.

Sprinkle with low sodium salt and pepper and toss to coat evenly.

Bake for 15-20 minutes until soft.

While the tomatoes are roasting, heat one tablespoon of olive oil in a large pan over low heat. Add the onions and mushrooms and cook for 10-12 minutes to soften and caramelize, stirring regularly. Clear a space for the chicken.

Season the turkey with low sodium salt and pepper and then place it in the pan.

Simmer for 15 minutes or until the chicken is cooked through. Every 5 minutes or so, spoon the sauce in the pan over the turkey.

To assemble, divide the tomatoes between two plates. Place one turkey breast on each and then spoon the onions, mushrooms, and pan drippings over the turkey. Garnish with parsley.

4. Sexy Turkey Scramble

Ingredients:
1 pound ground turkey
2 medium yellow onions
2 bell peppers (any color)
2 medium squash or zucchini
1 large hand-full of fresh spinach (2-3 ounces)
Spices to taste: I used about 1 tablespoon each of: cumin, chili powder, garlic powder, low sodium salt, and fresh cilantro

Instructions:
Brown the turkey until well cooked in a large skillet or wok over medium high heat.

Remove and add thinly sliced onions, peppers, squash/zucchini to the pan and saute, stirring constantly, until starting to soften.

Return turkey to pan and add fresh spinach.

Spice to taste and continue to cook until spinach is wilted.

Remove and serve with any desired toppings.

5. Sensational Courgette Pasta and Turkey Bolognese

Ingredients:
4 medium zucchini

For the sauce:
1 lb ground turkey
1 small onion, chopped
4 cloves garlic, minced
1 tbsp coconut oil
1 tomato, chopped
1/2 jar of tomato sauce
1 tbsp Italian seasoning
low sodium salt and pepper to taste
Fresh basil, for garnish

Instructions:
Use a julienne peeler to slice the zucchini into noodles, stopping when you reach the seeds. Set aside.

If cooking zucchini noodles, simply add to a skillet and sauté over medium heat for 4-5 minutes.

Melt coconut oil in a large skillet over medium heat. Add chopped onion and garlic and cook for 4-5 minutes.

Add ground turkey and brown the meat, stirring occasionally. Season with low sodium salt and pepper.

Add the chopped tomato, tomato sauce, and Italian seasoning and stir to combine. Simmer on low heat, stirring occasionally.

Add the sauce to the noodles and ENJOY.

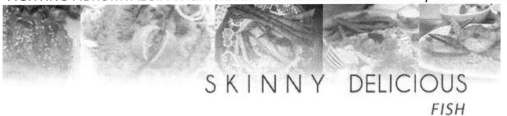

S K I N N Y   DELICIOUS
FISH

ANTI INFLAMMATORY Fish

1. Divine Prawn Mexicana

Ingredients:
1 tbsp extra virgin olive oil
1 tsp chili powder
1 tsp low sodium salt
1 lb. medium shrimp, peeled and deveined
1 avocado, pitted and diced
Shredded lettuce, for serving
Fresh cilantro, for serving
1 lime, cut into wedges

For the tortillas:
6 egg whites
1/4 cup coconut flour
1/4 cup almond milk
1/2 tsp low sodium salt
1/2 tsp cumin
1/4 tsp chili powder

Instructions:
Combine all of the tortilla ingredients together in a small bowl and mix well. Allow the batter to sit for approximately 10 minutes to allow the flour to soak up some of the moisture, and then stir again. The consistency should be similar to crepe batter.

While the batter is resting, heat a skillet to medium-high. Mix together the olive oil, chili powder, and low sodium salt and toss with the shrimp to coat.

Cook in the skillet for 1-2 minutes per side, until translucent. Set aside.

Coat the pan with coconut oil spray. Pour about 1/4 cup of batter onto the skillet, turning the pan with your wrist to help it spread out in a thin, even layer. Cook for 1-2 minutes, loosening the sides with a spatula. When the bottom has firmed up, carefully flip over and cook for another 2-3 minutes until lightly browned, then set aside on a plate.

Repeat with remaining batter.

Top each tortilla with cooked shrimp, shredded lettuce, avocado, and cilantro. Serve with a lime wedge.

2. Superior Salmon with Lemon and Thyme OR Use any White fish

Ingredients:
32 oz piece of salmon or any fresh white fish
1 lemon, sliced thin
1 tbsp capers
low sodium salt and freshly ground pepper
1 tbsp fresh thyme
Olive oil

Instructions:
Line a rimmed baking sheet with parchment paper and place salmon, skin side down, on the prepared baking sheet.

Season salmon with low sodium salt and pepper. Arrange capers on the salmon, and top with sliced lemon and thyme.

Place baking sheet in a cold oven, then turn heat to 400 degrees F. Bake for 25 minutes. Serve immediately.

3. Spectacular Shrimp Scampi in Spaghetti Sauce

Ingredients:
For the Spaghetti:
1 spaghetti squash
Extra virgin olive oil, for drizzling
low sodium salt and pepper
1 tsp dried oregano
1 tsp dried basil

For the shrimp scampi:
8 oz. shrimp, peeled and deveined
3 tbsp butter
1 tbsp extra virgin olive oil
2 cloves garlic, minced
Pinch of red pepper flakes
low sodium salt and pepper, to taste
1 tbsp fresh parsley, chopped
Juice of 1 lemon
Zest of half a lemon

Instructions:
Preheat the oven to 400 degrees F.

Place squash in the microwave for 3-4 minutes to soften.

Using a sharp knife, cut the squash in half lengthwise.

Scoop out the seeds and discard. Place the halves, with the cut side up, on a rimmed baking sheet.

Drizzle with olive oil and sprinkle with seasonings. Roast in the oven for 45-50 minutes, until you can poke the squash easily with a fork.

Let it cool until you can handle it safely. Then scrape the insides with a fork to shred the squash into strands.

After removing spaghetti squash from the oven, melt the butter and olive oil in a skillet over medium heat.

Add in the garlic and sauté for 2-3 minutes. Then add in the shrimp, low sodium salt, pepper, and a pinch of red pepper flakes.

Cook for 5 minutes, until the shrimp is cooked through.

Remove from heat and add in desired amount of cooked spaghetti squash.

Toss with lemon juice and zest.

Top with parsley.

4. Scrumptious Cod in Delish Sauce

Ingredients:
1 lb. cod fillets
1/3 cup almond flour
1/2 tsp low sodium salt
2-3 tbsp extra virgin olive oil
2 tbsp walnut oil, divided
3/4 cup low sodium chicken stock
3 tbsp lemon juice
1/4 cup capers, drained
2 tbsp fresh parsley, chopped

Instructions:
Stir the almond flour and low sodium salt together in a shallow bowl.

Rinse off the fish and pat dry with a paper towel. Dredge the fish in the almond flour mixture to coat.

Heat enough olive oil to coat the bottom of a large skillet over medium-high heat along with one tablespoon walnut oil. Working in batches, add the cod and cook for 2-3 minutes per side to brown. Remove to a plate and set aside.

Add the chicken stock, lemon juice, and capers to the same skillet and scrape any browned bits off the bottom. Simmer to reduce the sauce by almost half.

Remove from heat and stir in the remaining tablespoon of walnut oil.

To serve, divide the cod onto plates, drizzle with the sauce, and sprinkle with parsley.

5. Mouthwatering Stuffed Salmon

Ingredients:
1 lb wild Alaskan or sockeye salmon, cut into 2 pieces
6 oz raw shrimp, peeled, deveined and chopped
1 large egg
2 tbsp raw onions, chopped
2 tbsp Italian flat leaf parsley, chopped
2 tbsp almond meal (or almond flour)
2 tbsp coconut butter
1 clove garlic, minced
low sodium salt and pepper to taste

Instructions:
For the Salmon:
Preheat oven to 400F
Pat dry the salmon filets with a paper towel.
Combine the cinnamon, coriander, cumin, cloves, and cardamom. Sprinkle evenly over the salmon filet side.
Heat an oven safe skillet (preferably cast iron) to medium high heat. Test the heat by placing a drop of water. It should immediately evaporate.
Add the coconut butter and let it melt.
Place the salmon filet side down and let sear for about 1-2 minutes. Flip and sear on the skin side for 1 minute.
Place the skillet inside the oven, with the skin side down.
Bake at 400F for 6-7 minutes.

For the Lime Mustard Mayo:

Combine dressing, lime juice, low sodium salt, and mustard.

Dip with salmon and enjoy!

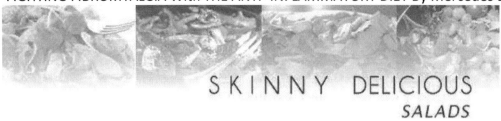

SKINNY DELICIOUS
SALADS

ANTI INFLAMMATORY Salads

1. Rosy Chicken Supreme Salad

Ingredients:
For the chicken:
450g chicken mince, free range of course
1 long red chili, finely chopped with the seeds
2 garlic cloves, finely chopped
Little nob of fresh ginger, peeled and finely chopped
1 stem lemon grass, pale section only, finely chopped
1/2 bunch of coriander stems washed and finely chopped (I don't waste anything, save the leaves for the salad)
2 1/2 tbsp fish sauce
1/2 lime rind grated
1/2 lime, juiced
A pinch of low sodium salt
Coconut oil for frying (about 3 tablespoons)

For the salad:
1/4 red cabbage, thinly sliced
1 large carrot, peeled and grated
1/2 Spanish onion, thinly sliced
2 tbsp green spring onion, chopped
1/2 bunch of fresh coriander leaves (saved from the stems used in the chicken)
A handful of fresh mint or Thai basil if available
1/2 cup crashed roasted cashews or some sesame seeds

For the dressing:
2 tbsp olive oil
3 tbsp lime juice
1 tbsp fish sauce

1 small red chili, finely chopped

Instructions:

Once you've prepared all your ingredients for the chicken, heat 1 tbsp of coconut oil in a large frying pan or a wok to high.

Throw in lemongrass, chili, garlic, coriander stems and ginger and stir fry for about a minute until fragrant.

Add chicken mince and lime zest. Stir and break apart the mince with a wooden mixing spoon until separated into small chunks (this might take a while as chicken mince is quite sticky).

The meat will now be changing to white colour.

Add fish sauce and lime juice. Stir through and cook for a further few minutes. Total cooking time for the chicken should be about 10 minutes.

Prepare the salad base by mixing together sliced red cabbage, onion grated carrot, and fresh herbs.

Mix all dressing ingredients and toss through the salad.

Serve cooked chicken mince on top of the dressed salad and topped with roasted cashews, dried shallots, coconut flakes and extra fresh herbs.

2. Sexy Italian Tuna Salad

Ingredients:
10 sun-dried tomatoes
2 (5 oz) can of tuna
1-2 ribs of celery, diced finely
2 Tablespoons of extra virgin olive oil
1 cloves garlic, minced
3 Tablespoons finely chopped parsley
1/2 Tablespoon lemon juice
low sodium salt and pepper to taste

Instructions:
Prepare the sun-dried tomatoes by softening them in warm water for 30 minutes until soft. Then, pat the tomatoes dry and chop finely.

Flake the tuna.

Mix the tuna together with the chopped tomatoes, celery, extra virgin olive oil, garlic, parsley, and lemon juice. Add low sodium salt and pepper to taste.

If not serving immediately, mix with extra olive oil just before serving.

Optional: Make cucumber boats with them.

3. Skinny Chicken salad

Ingredients:

Salad:
1 small head (or 4 cups) savoy cabbage, finely shredded –
1 cup carrot, julienned
1/4 cup scallions, trimmed and julienned
1/4 cup radishes, julienned
1/4 cup fresh cilantro, chopped
1/4 cup fresh mint, chopped
2 cups cooked organic chicken

Vinaigrette:
2 tablespoons coconut or rice vinegar
2 tablespoons sesame oil (use unrefined or cold-pressed)
juice of 1/2 a lime
1 chipotle pepper - optional
1 clove garlic, crushed
1 teaspoon fresh ginger, grated

Instructions:

Salad – Combine cabbage, carrots, scallions and radishes. Top with chicken, cilantro and mint and set aside.

Vinaigrette –Combine the vinaigrette ingredients. Taste to see if it needs any adjustments. If it is too spicy, you can add more lime juice to counteract it.

Drizzle salad with vinaigrette & enjoy.

4. Turkey Taco Salad

Ingredients:
1/2 lbs (ish) leftover turkey, cooked and chopped
1 1/2 Tbsp taco seasoning (recipe follows)
1 tblsp. coconut or olive oil and 1 tblsp rice vinegar
1/4 c. water
Shredded lettuce

Optional Toppings - sliced olives, tomatoes, red onion, avocado, bell peppers,
crushed sweet potato chips

Taco Seasoning:
Mix together, 4 Tbsp. chili powder, 1 tsp each garlic powder, onion powder, and oregano, 2 tsp each paprika and cumin, 4 tsp low sodium salt, and 1/8-1/4 tsp red pepper flakes.

Instructions:
In a skillet, heat 1 teaspoon oil and add in chicken - I like to fry it for a minute to give some extra flavor. Add in water and taco seasoning, let simmer until liquid is gone.

Meanwhile, shred, chop, and dice all your toppings.

Assemble, lettuce, optional toppings, chicken, leftover oil and vinegar dressing, and crushed chips.

5. Cheeky Turkey Salad

Ingredients:
For the Turkey:
1 lb boneless turkey breasts
1 tbsp olive oil
low sodium salt and pepper, to taste

For the Salsa:
1 large tomato, quartered
1/2 red onion, cut into large chunks
1 garlic clove, peeled
1 small bunch of cilantro leaves
Juice of 1 lime
low sodium salt and pepper, to taste

Instructions:
Preheat oven to 375 F.

Bake turkey breasts dipped in olive oil on a baking sheet for 35 to 40 minutes, until no longer pink in the center.

While baking, add all salsa ingredients to a food processor and pulse using the chopping blade until finely chopped. Transfer the salsa to a large bowl and clean out the food processor. You will be using it to shred the turkey.

(If you don't have a food processor, just dice the tomato, onion, pepper, cilantro and garlic and add to a bowl with the lime juice, low sodium salt and pepper).

Remove turkey from the oven and allow to cool. Once cool enough to handle, cut each breast into three or four smaller pieces and add to the food processor. Pulse using the chopping blade until shredded.

Add turkey to bowl with salsa and mix well with a fork.

Refrigerate for at least two hours until turkey salad is chilled.

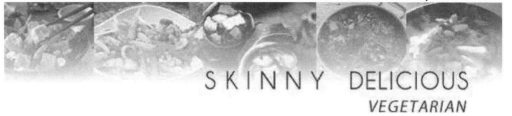

SKINNY DELICIOUS
VEGETARIAN

ANTI INFLAMMATORY Pure Vegetables

1. Rucola Salad

Ingredients:
4 teaspoons fresh lemon juice
4 teaspoons walnut oil
low sodium salt and freshly ground pepper
6 cups rucola leaves and tender stems (about 6 ounces)
Garlic powder to taste

Instructions:
Pour the lemon juice into a large bowl. Gradually whisk in the oil. Season with low sodium salt and pepper.

Add the greens, toss until evenly dressed and serve at once. This is delicious, and feel free to add tomatoes or grated carrot and onion slices.

Substitution: Any mild green, such as lamb's lettuce will do.

2. Tasty Spring Salad

Ingredients:
5 cups of any salad greens in season of your choice

Dressing:
125 mL (1/2 cup) olive oil
45 mL (3 tbsp) lemon juice
15 mL (1 tbsp) pure mustard powder
45 mL (3 tbsp) capers, minced (optional)
low sodium salt
pepper

Instructions:
Combine salad greens and any other raw vegetables of choice.

Combine oil, lemon juice and mustard. Mix well.

Add capers, low sodium salt and pepper to taste.

Pour dressing over salad, toss and serve.

3. Pure Delish Spinach Salad

Ingredients:
2 bunches fresh spinach
1 bunch scallions, chopped
juice of 1 lemon
1/4 tbsp olive oil
pepper to taste

optional: rice vinegar to taste

Instructions:
Wash spinach well. Drain and chop.

After a few minutes, squeeze excess water.

Add scallions, lemon juice, oil and pepper.

4. Sexy Salsa Salad

Ingredients:
1 bunch of cilantro
5-6 roma tomatoes
1 small yellow or red onion
1 small chili pepper
2 ripe avocados.
handful of rucola leaf

Instructions:
Chop cilantro, dice tomatoes, dice onion, finely dice chili pepper, dice avocado.

After dicing each ingredient add to large bowl. Add rucola to bowl.

When finished, toss.

5. Jalapeno Salsa

Ingredients:
1 jalapeno pepper seeded and chopped fine
2 large ripe tomatoes, peeled and chopped
1 medium onion, minced
2 tbsp olive oil
juice of 1 lemon
1/2 tsp dried oregano
pepper to taste

Instructions:
Combine all ingredients and mix well.

Refrigerate covered until ready to eat.

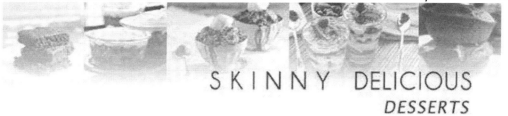

SKINNY DELICIOUS
DESSERTS

ANTI INFLAMMATORY Desserts

1. Fabulous Brownie Treats

Ingredients:
1 1/2 cups walnuts
Pinch of low sodium salt
1 tsp vanilla
1/3 cup unsweetened cocoa powder
Stevia to taste

Instructions:
Add walnuts and low sodium salt to a blender or food processor. Mix until the walnuts are finely ground.

Add the vanilla, and cocoa powder etc to the blender. Mix well until everything is combined.

With the blender still running, add a couple drops of water at a time to make the mixture stick together.

Using a spatula, transfer the mixture into a bowl. Using your hands, form small round balls, rolling in your palm.

2. Pristine Pumpkin Divine

Ingredients:
2 cups blanched almond flour
½ cup flaxseed meal
2 teaspoons ground cinnamon (optional)
Stevia to taste
½ teaspoon low sodium salt
1 egg
1 cup pumpkin puree
1 tablespoon vanilla extract

Instructions:
Mix together the almond flour, flaxseed meal, cinnamon, and low sodium salt

In a separate bowl, whisk the egg, pumpkin and vanilla extract using a rubber spatula.

Gently mix dry and wet ingredients to form a batter being careful not to over mix or the batter will get oily and dense.

Spoon the batter onto a 9-inch pan lined with parchment paper or grease the pan

bake at 350°F until a toothpick inserted into the center comes out clean, approximately 25 minutes.

FIGHTING FIBROMYALGIA With THE ANTI- INFLAMMATORY DIET By Mercedes Del Rey

3. Spectacular Spinach Brownies

Ingredients:
1 ¼ cups frozen chopped spinach
6 oz sugar free chocolate
½ cup extra virgin coconut oil
½ cup coconut oil
6 eggs
Stevia to taste
½ cup cocoa powder
1 Tspn vanilla pod
¼ tsp baking soda
½ tsp low sodium salt
½ tsp cream of tartar
pinch cinnamon

Instructions:
Preheat oven to 325F. Line a 9"x13" baking pan with wax paper or use a silicone baking pan.

Melt coconut oil and chocolate together over low heat on the stove top or medium power in the microwave. Add vanilla and stir to incorporate. Let cool.

Mix cocoa powder, baking soda, cream of tartar, low sodium salt and cinnamon.

Blend spinach, egg, together in a food processor or blender, until completely smooth (2-4 minutes).

Add coconut oil to food processor and process until full incorporated.

Add melted chocolate mixture and 3 or 4 drops stevia liquid to egg mixture slowly and processing/blending constantly.

Mix in dry ingredients and process/stir to fully incorporate.

Pour batter into prepared baking pan and spread out with a spatula.

Bake for 40 minutes. Cool completely in pan. Cut into squares. Enjoy!

4. Chestnut- Cacao Cake

Ingredients:
100g (1 cup + 1 heaping tablespoon) chestnut flour
50g (1/2 cup) ground almonds (almond flour)
3 eggs, separate
1/2 teaspoon cream of tartar
35g (1/2 cup) raw cacao powder
Stevia to taste
3/4 cup coconut milk
1/2 teaspoon baking soda
Crushed chestnuts

Instructions:
Preheat oven to 180C fan (350F).

Grease a pie/tart pan.

In a clean mixing bowl, beat the egg whites and cream of tartar until stiff peaks form. Set aside.

In another mixing bowl, cream the egg yolks, chestnut flour, ground almonds, stevia, raw cacao, baking soda and coconut milk.

Fold in the egg whites and blend until the white is no longer showing.

Pour into the pie/tart mold.

Sprinkle with crushed chestnuts, if desired.

Bake for 35-40 minutes on the middle rack.

5. Choco Cookie Delight

Ingredients:
1/2 cup dark chocolate sugar free chips
1/2 cup coconut milk (thick fat from top of can)
2 eggs
1 cup almond flour
pinch of low sodium salt
1/2 teaspoon vanilla extract
1/4 teaspoon baking powder

Vanilla glaze:
1/2 cup coconut butter, liquid
Stevia to taste
1 /2 teaspoon vanilla extract

Chocolate Glaze:
1/2 cup chocolate chips
Stevia powder for decoration

Instructions:
Place a small sauce pan over low heat and melt your chocolate and coconut milk together (only keep the heat on long enough to melt them together)

While melting, place your 2 eggs in a stand mixer with the whisk, or use a hand mixer with the whisk and beat your eggs until they are fluffy, about 1 minute

Add your coconut milk and chocolate to your eggs and mix well

Stir in your almond flour, low sodium salt, vanilla extract and baking powder

Mix well ensuring everything is combined

Pipe your batter into the cookie wells ensuring you fill higher than the halfway point

Remove from the cookie maker, gently insert the sticks and place everything in the freezer for 30-45 minutes

Vanilla Glaze:

Combine your coconut butter, stevia, and vanilla extract in a small glass to make it easy to dip

You can keep this glass in hot water to keep the glaze more liquidy to make the dipping easier

Chocolate Glaze:

Melt your chocolate chips over a double boiler and keep the heat low and them liquid – then spread over cooled cookies!

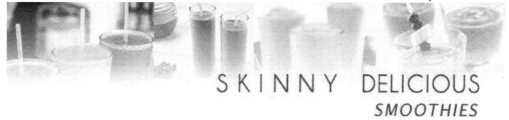

SKINNY DELICIOUS
SMOOTHIES

ANTI INFLAMMATORY Smoothies

1. Voluptuous Vanilla Hot Drink

Ingredients:
3 cups unsweetened almond milk (or 1 1/2 cup full fat coconut milk + 1 1/2 cups water)
Stevia to taste
1 scoop of hemp protein
1/2 Tbsp. ground cinnamon (or more to taste)
1/2 Tbsp. vanilla extract

Instructions:
Place the almond milk into a pitcher. Place ground cinnamon, hemp, vanilla extract in a small saucepan over medium high heat. Heat until the pure liquid stevia is just melted and then pour the pure liquid stevia mixture into the pitcher.

Stir until the pure liquid stevia is well combined with the almond milk. Place the pitcher in the fridge and allow to chill for at least two hours. Stir well before serving.

2. Almond Butter Smoothies

Ingredients:
1 scoop of hemp protein
1 Tablespoon natural almond butter
1 cup of hemp milk
1 banana, preferably frozen for a creamier shake
few ice cubes

Instructions:
Blend all ingredients together and enjoy!

3. Baby Kale Pineapple Smoothie

Ingredients:
1 cup almond milk
1/2 cup frozen pineapple
1 cup Kale
1 tablespoon hemp protein powder

Instructions:
Place the almond milk, pineapple, and greens in the blender and blend until smooth.

4. Vanilla Blueberry Smoothie

Ingredients:
2 cups hemp milk
1 c fresh blueberries
Handful of ice OR 1 cup frozen blueberries
1 Tbsp flaxseed oil
2 tblsp hemp protein powder

Instructions:
Combine milk, and fresh blueberries plus ice (or frozen blueberries) in a blender.

Blend for 1 minute, transfer to a glass, and stir in flaxseed oil.

5. Zesty Citrus Smoothie

Ingredients:
1 cup almond milk
half cup lemon juice
1 med orange peeled, cleaned, and sliced into sections
Handful of ice
1 Tbsp flaxseed oil
2 tsp hemp protein powder

Instructions:
COMBINE milk, lemon juice, orange, and ice in a blender.

Blend for 1 minute, transfer to a glass, and stir in flaxseed oil.

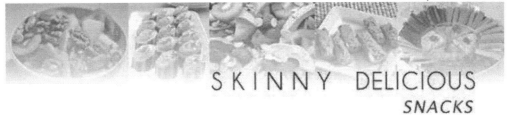

SKINNY DELICIOUS
SNACKS

ANTI INFLAMMATORY Snacks

1. Delectable Parsnip Chips

Ingredients:
500g (1.1 pounds) Parsnips
1/4 Cup Coconut Oil, Melted
3 Tablespoons liquid stevia

Instructions:
Preheat the oven to 200°C (392°F) and get out an oven proof dish.

Peel the parsnips and cut them into chip sized pieces and place into the oven proof dish.

Pour over the coconut oil and distribute evenly.

Drizzle over the liquid stevia and stir to combine well.

Place in the oven and cook for 15 minutes.

Remove from the oven and toss the parsnips over to allow the other side to brown.

Place back in the oven and cook for a further 10 to 15 minutes or until golden.

2. Skinny Power Snack

Ingredients:
1/2 Avocado
1/2 tsp Paprika
1/2 tsp low sodium salt
1/2 tsp Garlic Powder

Instructions:
Sprinkle with all the seasonings and enjoy.

3. Gummy Citrus Snack

Ingredients:
3/4 cup lemon juice, freshly squeezed*
¼ cup apple juice freshly squeezed
4 Tbsp. good quality vegetarian gelatin
liquid stevia to taste
1/4 tsp. ginger (freshly grated or ground)
1/4 tsp. turmeric (freshly grated or ground)

Instructions:
In a small saucepan, whisk together citrus juice, and gelatin until there are no lumps. Heat the liquid over low heat until liquid is warmed and gelatin is completely dissolved.

Remove from heat and stir in liquid stevia, ginger and turmeric with a spoon.

Pour into a casserole dish*.

Refrigerate until liquid is set (at least 30 minutes).

Serve cold or at room temperature.

4. Gorgeous Spicy Nuts

Ingredients:
2/3 cup of each (almonds, pecans and walnuts)
1 teaspoon of chili powder
½ teaspoon of cumin
½ teaspoon of black
pepper (ground)
½ teaspoon low sodium salt
1 tables

Instructions:
Heat the pan on medium heat and place the nuts and toast them until lightly browned.

Prepare the spice mixture, while the nuts are toasting.

Mix cumin, chili, low sodium salt and black pepper in a bowl and add the nuts (after coating it with olive oil).

5. Spicy Pumpkin Seed Bonanza

Ingredients:
1 1/2 cups pumpkin seeds,
3 jalapeño peppers, sliced
3 tablespoons olive oil
low sodium salt and paprika, to taste

Instructions:
Preheat the oven to 350°F

Spread pumpkin seeds out on a rimmed baking sheet.

Add olive oil and low sodium salt and stir pumpkin seeds with your hands to combine.

Lay slices of jalapeño peppers on top of seeds.

Sprinkle paprika over the top of everything, generously.

Bake for 10 minutes.

Use a spatula to move the seeds and peppers around. Bake for another 5 minutes.

Move mixture around some more and bake for a final 5 minutes.

Remove tray from oven and let everything rest for 15-30 minutes to let the jalapeño-ness soak into the seeds.

Store in an airtight container...if you don't finish them all in one sitting.

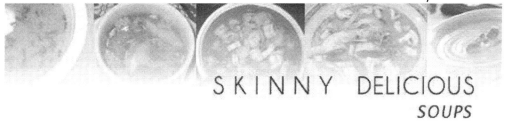

S K I N N Y DELICIOUS

SOUPS

ANTI INFLAMMATORY Soups

1. Cheeky Chicken Soup

Ingredients:
2 large organic chicken breasts, skin removed and cut into ½ inch strips
1 28oz can of diced tomatoes
32 ounces low sodium organic chicken broth
1 sweet onion, diced
2 cups of shredded carrots
2 cups chopped celery
1 bunch of cilantro chopped fine
4 cloves of garlic, minced - I always use one of these
2 Tbs tomato paste
1 tsp chili powder
1 tsp cumin
low sodium salt & fresh cracked pepper to taste
olive oil
1-2 cups water

Instructions:
In a crockpot place a dash of olive oil and about ¼ cup chicken broth. Add onions, garlic, jalapeno, low sodium salt and pepper and cook until soft, adding more broth as needed.

Then add all of your remaining ingredients and enough water to fill to the top of your pot. Cover and let cook on low for about 2 hrs, adjusting low sodium salt & pepper as needed.

Once the chicken is fully cooked, you should be able to shred it very easily. I simply used the back of a wooden spoon and pressed the cooked chicken against the side of the pot.

Top with avocado slices and fresh cilantro. Enjoy!

2. Ginger Carrot Delight Soup

Ingredients:

3 tbsp unsalted butter or coconut oil
1 1/2 pounds carrots (6-7 large carrots), sliced
2 cups chopped white or yellow onion
1 cup diced turkey breast
low sodium salt
2 teaspoons minced ginger
2 cups low sodium chicken stock
2 cups water
3 large strips of zest from an orange

Instructions:

Heat up the butter or coconut oil in a large soup pot.

Add the chopped carrots, turkey breast and onion to the pot and cook over medium heat for 5-10 minutes. Don't allow the carrots or onion to brown.

Add in the remaining ingredients (ginger, orange zest, water, and stock). The orange zest will be pulled out prior to puréeing so make sure they are in large, easy to identify strips rather than small pieces.

Bring to a boil then simmer for 10 minutes.

Remove orange zest strips.

Purée the mixture with an immersion blender. Or divide into 3-4 batches and blend in a regular blender.

I garnished my soup with a touch of olive oil and some freshly ground low sodium salt and pepper.

FIGHTING FIBROMYALGIA With THE ANTI- INFLAMMATORY DIET By Mercedes Del Rey

3. Wonderful Watercress Soup

Ingredients:
1 quart low sodium chicken stock
1 medium leek
1 bunch water cress
1 large onion
1/2 celeriac root skinned and chopped
2 cups diced chicken breast - organic
low sodium salt and pepper to taste

Instructions:
Gently heat the chicken stock in the pot.

In the fry pan sauté the onion, leek and celeriac until soft.

Place the onion, leek, chicken and celeriac in the pot of stock reserving 1/3 aside.

Season with low sodium salt and pepper.

Add the bunch of watercress and simmer a few minutes until it is wilted.

With the immersion blender blend the soup.

Add the chopped vegetables that you reserved, back into the pot.

4. Celery Cashew Cream Soup

Ingredients:
300 grams celery, washed and chopped
1 small onion, chopped
1.5 tbsp olive oil
500 mls vegetable stock
40 grams cashew nuts
low sodium salt and pepper to taste

Instructions:
Heat the olive oil in a large saucepan then add the celery and onion, stir to coat with oil. Turn the heat low and put the lid on leaving the vegetables to sweat for 5 minutes.

Add the garlic, give a quick stir then add the vegetable stock and simmer for 10 minutes.

Add the cashew nuts to the saucepan and simmer for another 5 minutes or until the celery is cooked through.

Tip the soup mix into a blender and purée until smooth.

Season with the low sodium salt and pepper and serve.

5. Mighty Andalusian Gazpacho

Ingredients:
3 pounds very ripe tomatoes, cored and cut into chunks
½ pound cucumber, peeled, seeded, and cut chunks
⅓ pound red onion, peeled and cut into chunks
⅓ pound green or red bell pepper, cored, seeded, and cut into chunks
2 cloves garlic, peeled and smashed
1½ teaspoons low sodium salt, plus more to taste
1 cup extra-virgin olive oil, plus more for serving
2 tablespoons sherry vinegar, plus more for serving
2 tablespoons finely minced chives
Freshly ground black pepper

Instructions:
Put all veggies in a large bowl and toss with low sodium salt. Let sit till the veggies have released a lot of their liquid.

Separate the veggies from the liquid, reserving the liquid. Place on a tray and place in the freezer for at least a half hour, or until they are partially frozen.

Remove from freezer and let thaw completely.

Combine the thawed veggies, reserved juice, oil and sherry vinegar in a large bowl. Ladle into a blender, working in batches if necessary, and blend on high until quite smooth. Chill for up to 24 hours.

Serve with extra sherry vinegar, olive oil and a sprinkle of chives

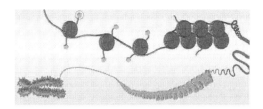

Chapter 15

The ANTI INFLAMMATORY Vision

We've covered some very important ground so far in identifying the best ways to get you to the healthier, leaner, genetically smarter new you. Epigenetics prove in the clearest possible terms that we can influence and control our bodies at every level by taking control of what we eat and how we behave.

We've introduced you to the key points in your action plan for weight loss control and opened up a whole new world of health and wellbeing possibilities. But we have another important insight to share with you. And now is the perfect moment to reveal it!

Humans have a secret weapon in their behavioural armoury that can work powerfully to help us - or it can work just as powerfully against us. It's our imagination. Or rather it's our ability to visualise. Most of the time, our thoughts drift around in a random pattern of uncoordinated ideas, prompted by whatever happens to pop up around us. We are drawn to whatever grabs our fickle attention.

Our thoughts and feelings are largely conditioned from early childhood experiences that shape our future emotional framework. We learn from an early age to let our thoughts pretty much wander wherever they choose. The mind follows random currents, blown around like a leaf in the wind, lacking focus or any sense of direction. A ship without a rudder.

This is where the risks of self-sabotage emerge; uncontrolled thoughts and feelings, self-doubt, memories of failure, feelings of a lack of self-worth. The list is endless and potentially destructive to our plans for absolute wellbeing. So now is the perfect time to switch on our powers of visualisation and give the mind some clear directions to follow for the future. It's time to bring on the really powerful support system that is hidden within your own mind!

FIGHTING FIBROMYALGIA With THE ANTI- INFLAMMATORY DIET By Mercedes Del Rey

It's incredible to realise how much our expectations shape our perceptions and our behaviour. Our programmed attitudes and responses play a major role in determining many of the outcomes in our lives. Happily, humans possess the immensely powerful gift of visualisation.

By visualising a desired outcome, our behaviours shift to favour those clearly visualised results. The technique of visualisation is incredibly simple. All we have to do is relax. That's right. Relax. Sit down and relax and close your eyes. Now breathe a little more deeply. And see yourself exactly as you really, deeply desire yourself to be.

See your smiling face, see each part of your radiantly healthy, skinnier new body. Smile at the strength, health, energy and vitality that surges through your newly visualised body. And feel really happy about it. Underline the vision with a warm, happy feeling of complete wellbeing. Hold the picture and imagine taking a photograph with your mind. Hear the camera shutter click as you record the stunning new picture of how you are. The picture of who you are becoming.

The powerful vision of the happier, fitter, skinnier new you! Lock this picture in your mind. Hold it in your heart. See it every time you close your eyes. This vision is the future. Use it all the time and you will rally all your hidden creative resources to bring this beautiful new vision of yourself into being.

We do not live in a culture that highlights the importance of mindfulness. We are constantly bombarded by images, noises, distractions and background chaos. We also have to live with the judgement of everyone around us. No wonder we find it difficult to concentrate and to relax. But there are many, simple and effective methods that can help us train our minds to follow our directions and meditation probably offers the simplest, most obvious and direct advantages. There is no religious or philosophical aspect to this exercise. It's just a technique for calming the mind. It takes only fifteen minutes. But it's a method that requires fifteen minutes every day. The daily repetition amplifies the results.

The only equipment you need is a chair, preferably a firm chair with good support for your back. A straight back is supposed to be better for meditation. Being comfortable is also very helpful. Relax your hands on your lap, close your eyes, focus on the spot between your eyebrows and breathe. Just follow your breath gently in and out. That's it. No chanting, humming or repeating strange mantras.

Just good old-fashioned breathing and the focus of concentrating lightly on the breath. The effects are cumulative. They build up gradually as you practise every day. You'll feel calmer. You'll find your powers of concentration improve. You'll be able to relax more easily. Your power to visualise will become more sharply defined. Your mind will begin to follow your directions. You will get a sense of the potential within you. Mastering the mind is a method for mastering ourselves. All this from just fifteen minutes a day. The effects might surprise you because as you learn to become calmer, your body will feel much more comfortable. No prescriptions are required. Just those simple fifteen minutes of daily meditation and you'll soon be looking forward to the sessions with real enthusiasm. You might enjoy the benefits so much that you'll want to meditate for longer.

FIGHTING FIBROMYALGIA With THE ANTI- INFLAMMATORY DIET By Mercedes Del Rey

Your vision of the happier, fitter, leaner, genetically smarter new you is the new background picture of your life. It represents the possibility of achieving everything you have chosen for yourself. Every day, you are living the journey of moving towards that possibility. The vision does not have a deadline. There can be no disappointment with the results because you are living every day in the possibility of its realisation.

Even if you slip and go backwards, the vision will put you back on track, guiding you every day towards its fulfillment. That's a powerful tool to have at your disposal. Put it to work right now. Use it every day. Use it every time you close your eyes and see the vision of how you are transforming yourself.

Ultimately, it's our behaviour that will guide our choices. Meditation is rightly considered to be a very powerful technique for bringing gentle control into the chaos of our minds. As we become more aware of our choices, as we experience the benefits of mindfulness, we can detect old patterns of behaviour that no longer fit our vision of health and vitality. We can understand the advantages of better choices.

We begin to respect the body's needs from a deeper, more caring perspective. The vision represents who we are becoming. The daily meditation helps us to become calmer, more resistant to stress and this healthier emotional framework lends itself to a physically healthier body. We also recommend a short meditation before you go to sleep at night. It's another effective way to calm the mind, still the thoughts and prepare for truly restful sleep.

Meditation has been practised as a tool for managing and directing the mind for thousands of years. It's so effective because we've been using it and refining the techniques as a species for millennia. We've highlighted the fundamental method here because we already use a form of meditation all the time. Have you noticed how easy it can be to day-dream? To drift off into another world of memories or fantasies, oblivious of what's happening around you? A brief reverie or a moment when you lose focus on what's going on around you?

These are altered states of consciousness and they happen all the time. Our purpose with the super simple meditation method is to control that tendency and direct it towards a focused, positive outcome. A way to become mindful yet relaxed. Aware yet calm. Centered yet connected. Still but alive with nurturing, positive energy. And all from fifteen minutes a day! Sounds like the bargain of a lifetime and it's all yours. For now and for the rest of your life.

You've heard it before and you're about to hear it again. We Are What We Eat. There's no getting away from it. You've learned enough by now to understand the vital connection between what you eat and how your body looks. Putting garbage into your body will ruin it. Eat garbage and you'll look like sh.., I mean, waste products. But you know this. That's why you've joined us on this mission of personal transformation.

So far we've been exploring the mechanics of healthy weight control, shedding unwanted pounds and promoting the best health we can possibly enjoy and we fully appreciate the importance of intelligent nutrition. But there are other challenges out there and we've hinted at some of them earlier in Chapter..... We're talking toxins, my friend. Those totally unfriendly substances that pollute our food, poison our drinks and surround us in the air we breathe. Our world has become a scarily toxic place to exist and most of the problems are man-made. That doesn't make them any easier to live with.

You already know how important it is to avoid toxins by eating as naturally as possible but what about the toxins we inhale? What about the poisons that leach into our skin from the environment? The answer to this problem and the best the way to give your body a fair chance to neutralise these poisons is to use a cleansing diet for a few days. Fresh vegetables are the easiest and best source of natural cleansing. They promote natural digestion and contain nutrients that are very helpful in maintaining your health and wellbeing.

Stick to the PALEO meal selection of the Epigenetic diet for a few days and you'll be amazed at the difference you'll feel in your overall wellness. And drink plenty of water too. The idea of cleansing the body is hardly new. We're just too busy to think of it. But now that we're on a journey of total physical transformation, let's give our bodies the best chance to feel fantastic.

And that means flushing out the garbage to restore total health and wellbeing. Getting away to a place with fresh air is another helpful way to restore balance to your body. Just breathing - and meditating - in the fresh air can work wonders for our health and vitality. Sea air, mountain air, the fresh air in the forest or open countryside can restore you at so many levels. If it's at all possible, make a regular date for a mini cleanse and for some valuable down time in the fresh, open air.

 Get a little help from your friends.

You're not alone. It's all too easy to imagine that we're the only ones who are experiencing problems, and think that the rest of the world is having fun, eating well and enjoying life to the full. But most of the world just isn't like that. Sharing your experiences, your challenges and difficulties, sharing your goals and intentions can gather support from everyone around you. You'll be surprised how many people will offer their encouragement and enthusiasm for your new way of life. It will help to reinforce your personal commitment to a healthier, fitter and happier way of being. So feel free to share and build that beautiful support group.

Personal Vision - Summary

Engaging the power of visualisation

Meditating on the powerful new you

Building a clear picture of who you are becoming

Daring to dream and engaging the power of focused visualisation

Total health and well being

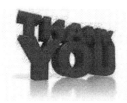

I am so delighted that you have chosen this book and it's been a pleasure writing it for you. My mission is to help as many readers as possible to benefit from the content you have just been reading. So many of us are able to take new information and apply it to our lives with really positive and long lasting consequences and it is my wish that you have been able to take value from the information I have presented.

Thank you for staying with me during this book and for reading it through to the end. I really hope that you have enjoyed the contents and that's why I appreciate your feedback so much. If you could take a couple of minutes to review the book, your views will help me to create more material that you find beneficial.

I am always delighted to hear from my readers and you can email me via the publisher at beranparry@gmail.com if you have any questions about this book or future books. Let us know how we can help you by sending a message to the same email address.

Thanks again for your support and encouragement. I really look forward to reading your review.

Stay Healthy!

References

Scientific Studies General

Boling, C. L., E. C. Westman, W. S. Yancy Jr. "Carbohydrate-Restricted Diets for Obesity and Related Diseases: An Update." *Current Atherosclerosis Reports* 11.6 (2008): 462-9.

Cahill, G. F., Jr. "Fuel Metabolism in Starvation." *Annual Review of Nutrition* 26 (2006): 1-22.

Feinman, R. D., M. Makowske. "Metabolic Syndrome and Low-Carbohydrate Ketogenic Diets in the Medical School Biochemistry Curriculum." *Metabolic Syndrome and Related Disorders* 1.3 (2003): 189-197.

Liu, Y. M. "Medium-Chain Triglyceride (MCT) Ketogenic Therapy." *Epilepsia* 49.Suppl 8 (2008): 33-6.

Manninen, A. H. "Is a Calorie Really a Calorie, Metabolic Advantage of Low-Carbohydrate Diets." *Journal of the International Society of Sports Nutrition* 1.2 (2004): 21-6.

McClernon, F. J., et al "The Effects of Low-Carbohydrate Ketogenic Diet and a Low-Fat on Mood, hunger and Other Self Reported Symptoms." *Obesity* (Silver Spring) 15.1 (2007): 182-7.

Paoli, A., A. Rubini, J. S. Volek, K. A. Grimaldi. "Beyond Weight Loss: A Review of the Therapeutic Uses of Very-Low-Carbohydrate (Ketogethc) Diets." *European Journal of Clinical Nutrition* 67 (2013): 789-796.

Veech, R. L. "The Therapeutic Implications of Ketone Bodies: The Effects of Ketone Bodies in Pathological Conditions: Ketosis, Ketogenic Diet, Redox States, Insulin Resistance, and Mitochondrial Metabolism." *Prostaglandins, Leukotrienes and Essential Fatty Acids* 70.3 (2004): 309-19.

Veech, R. L., et al. "Ketone Bodies, Potential Therapeutic Uses." *IUBMB Life* 51 (2001): 241-7.

Volek, J. S., C. E. Forsythe. "The Case for Not Restricting Saturated Fat on a Low Carbohydrate Diet." *Nutrition and Metabolism 2* (2005) :21.

Volek, J. S., C. E. Forsythe. "Very-Low-Carbohydrates ." *In Essentials of Sports Nutrition and Supplements*, edited by Jose Antonio, Douglas Kalman, Jeffrey R. Stout, Mike Greenwood, Darryn S. Willoughby, and G. Gregory H., 581-604. Totowa, NJ: Humana Press, 2008.

Moore, Jimmy, and Dr. Eric Westman. *Cholesterol Clarity: What the HDL Is Wrong with My Numbers?* Las Vegas, NV: Victory Belt Publishing, 2013. Newport, Dr. Mary. *Alzheimer's Disease: What If There Was Cure? The Story of Ketones*. Laguna Beach, CA: Basic Health Publications, 2011.

Ottoboni, Dr. Fred, and Dr. Alice Ottoboni. *The Modern Nutritional Disease: and How to Prevent Them*, Second Edition. Femly, NV: Vincente Books, 2013.

FIGHTING FIBROMYALGIA With THE ANTI- INFLAMMATORY DIET By Mercedes Del Rey

Perlmutter, Dr. David. Grain Brain: *The Surprising Truth about Wheat, Carbs, and Sugar-Your Brain, Silent Killers.* New York: Little, Brown, 2013.

Phinney, Dr. Stephen, and Dr. Jeff Volek. *The Art and Science of Low Carbohydrate Living*, Beyond Obesity, 2011.

Phinney, Dr. Stephen, and Dr. Jeff Volek. *The Art and Science of Low Carbohydrate Performance*. Beyond Obesity, 2012.

Seyfried, Dr. Thomas. *Cancer as a Metabolic Disease: On the Origin, Management, and Prevention of Cancer.* Hoboken, NJ: John Wiley & Sons, 2012.

Skaldeman, Sten Sture. *The Low Carb High Fat Cookbook:100 Recipes to Lose Weight and Feel Great.* New York: Skyhorse Publishing, 2013.

Snyder, Dr. Deborah. *Keto Kid: Helping Your Child Succeed on the Ketogenic Diet.* New York: Demos Medical Publishing, 2006.

Taubes, Gary. *Good Calories, Bad Calories: Challenging the Conventional Wisdom on Diet, Weight Control, and Disease.* New York: Anchor Books, 2007.

Taubes, Gary. *Why We Get Fat: And What to Do About It.* New York: Anchor Books, 2011.

Tiecholz, Tina. *The Big Fat Surprise: Why Butte, Meat, and Cheese Belong in a Healthy Diet.* New York: Simon 8. Schuster, 2014.

Volek, Dr. Jeff and Adam Campbell. *Men's Health TNT Diet: The Explosive New Plan to Blast Fat, Build Muscle, and Get Healthy in 12 Weeks.* New York Rodale, 2008

Wahls, Dr. Terry, and Eve Adamson. *The Wahls Protocol: How I Beat Progreuive MS Using Paleo Principles and Functional Medicine.* New York: Penguin, 2014.

Westman, Dr. Eric. *A Low Carbohydrate, Ketogenic Diet Manual, No Sugar, No Starch Diet.* Dr. Eric Westman, 2013.

Westman, Dr. Eric, Dr. Stephen D. Phinney, and Dr. Jeff S. Volek. *The New Atkins for a New You.* New York: Fireside, 2010.

Keto Slogs and Websites

Everything About Keto, Reddit: www.reddit.com/r/

keto Ketogenic Diet Resource: www.ketogenic-diet-resource.com

The Charlie Foundation for Ketogenic Therapies: www.charliefoundation.org

Anderson, W. (2009) The Anderson Method: The Secret to Permanent Weight Loss. Minneapolis: Two Harbors Press.

Arem, R. (2012) The Protein Boost Diet. New York: Atria Books.

Baird, J. (2012) Obesity Genes and their Epigenetic Modifiers. Naperville IL: HWL, Inc.

Bouchard, C. (2010) Genes and Obesity, Volume 94 (Progress in Molecular Biology & Translational Science). Burlington MA: Academic Press- Elsevier Inc.

Campbell, T and Campbell, T.C. (2006) The China Study: The Most Comprehensive Study of Nutrition Ever Conducted And the Startling Implications for Diet, Weight Loss, and Long-term Health. Dallas, TX: BenBella Books.

Campbell-Mc-Bride, N. (2010) Gut and Psychology Syndrome: Natural Treatment for Autism, Dyspraxia, A.D.D., Dyslexia, A.D.H.D., Depression, Schizophrenia. Amazon Digital Services, Inc. [10 June 2014].

Carey, N. (2012) The Epigenetics Revolution: How Modern Biology is Rewriting Our Understanding of Genetics, Disease and Inheritance. London: Icon Books Ltd.

Chopra, D. (2013) What are you Hungry For?: The Chopra Solution to Permanent Weight Loss, Well-Being, and Lightness of Soul. New York: Harmony Books.

Cordain, P. (2011) The Paleo Diet Revised Edition. New Jersey: John Wiley & Sons, Inc.

Dean, C. (2006) The Magnesium Miracle. New York: Ballantine Books; Updated Edition.

Ecker, S. (2014) Eating Well: How to build good eating habits to have your perfect body and overcome eating disorder. Available from: Amazon Digital Services, Inc. [2 September 2014].

Holick, M. (2011) The Vitamin D Solution: A 3-Step Strategy to Cure our Most Common Health Problems. New York: Hudson Street Press.

Kushner, L. et al. (2013) Practical Manual of Clinical Obesity. Chichester, West Sussex: John Wiley & Sons, Ltd.

Lask, B. (2011) Eating Disorders and the Brain. Oxford: Wiley-Blackwell.

Minger, D. (2014) Death by Food Pyramid: How Shoddy Science, Sketchy Politics, and Shady Special Interests Have Ruined Our Health…and How to Reclaim it! Malibu, CA: Primal Blueprint Publishing.

Power, M. and Schulkin, J. (2009) The Evolution of Obesity. Baltimore, MD: The Johns Hopkins University Press.

Sisson, M. (2013) The Primal Blueprint: Reprogram your genes for effortless weight loss, vibrant health, and boundless energy. Malibu, CA: Primal Nutrition, Inc.

Tollefsbol, T. (2014) Transgenerational Epigenetics. Waltham, MA: Academic Press- Elsevier Inc.

FREE BONUS CHAPTER

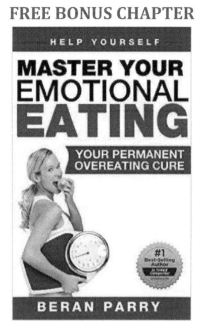

FROM THE MASTER YOUR EMOTIONAL EATING BOOK at

www.amazon.com/gp/product/B00UZP82QO?ie=UTF8&camp=1789&creativeASIN=B00UZP82QO&linkCode=xm2&tag=onelifeblog-20

How Does EMOTIONAL EATING Really Work?

We need to start with a very important question. Are you ready for it? Here it is: "Why do we feel out of control?" The answers are very important to our understanding of how to introduce change to our eating habits. We feel out of control when we doubt themselves, when we feel frustrated, when we feel vulnerable or unsafe, when we feel rebellious or angry, when we feel empty, when we feel unexpressed and, finally, when we feel unfulfilled.

When a person crosses over the threshold between using food as a source of sustenance and food as a source of comfort, that is the moment when food easily becomes a psychological support instead of a biological necessity. Whilst we cannot always pinpoint why this might have happened, this book will help you to examine in depth your own unique responses in each of the categories and help you to be finally free of this pattern of unhealthy eating behaviour.

FIGHTING FIBROMYALGIA With THE ANTI- INFLAMMATORY DIET By Mercedes Del Rey

In the first part of the book, you'll be able to understand and interpret the insights to discover action you need to take to achieve real and enduring change.

Then, in part two, you'll learn about each of these fascinating steps and how they've been affecting specific areas of your life.

Together we'll remove each of the barriers and obstacles as you set sail on your personal emotional eating journey of discovery. And I'll be with you to help, encouraging and coaching you to free the real you that's been hiding for too long behind your emotionally-driven behaviour.

We'll look at why, after so many efforts to be free of uncontrolled eating, you're still at a place where you feel utterly lost. But don't worry. You'll certainly be able to begin again – this time with a renewed sense of expectation, realization and partnership. As you strip away each of the barriers, your emotional dependence on food will diminish until one day you will look back with wonder and ask yourself why you needed all that food in the first place!

Emotional Eating can be very well described via the following statements:

We eat to suppress our feelings of fear, guilt, resentment, worry, irritation etc.

We chose comfort food like cakes and biscuits and sweets because we felt we needed/deserved it and then felt guilty about it.

We ate badly to punish our bodies for some imagined failure in our lives.

This is a great moment to work through a simple quiz to determine whether you are in fact an emotional eater or someone who uses food to cope with the stresses of life.

Are You an Emotional Eater?

To find out if you're an emotional eater, answer the following five questions.

The last time you ate too much

1.   When you needed to eat, did you feel a desperate and urgent need to eat something right away?

2.   When you ate, did you enjoy the taste of every bite, or did you just stuff it in?

3.   When you got hungry, did you need a certain type of food to satisfy yourself?

4.   Did you feel guilty after you ate the same day or the next day?

5.   Did you eat when you were emotionally upset or feeling that you "deserved" it

Let's see how you did.

194

1.   Physical hunger begins slowly, then it becomes a stronger and finally it evolves into hunger pangs, but it's a slow process, very different from emotional hunger, which has a sense of urgency

2.   There is a major difference between physical hunger and emotional hunger and it involves a degree of awareness. To satisfy physical hunger you normally make a deliberate choice about what you eat and you maintain awareness whilst you're eating. If you have emotional hunger, you won't notice how much you are eating or the taste and you will still want more food even after you're full.

3.   Emotional hunger often demands very specific foods in order to be fulfilled. If you're physically hungry, even a salad will look delicious. If you're emotionally hungry, however, only your specific and possibly toxic choice will seem appealing.

4.   Emotional eating often results in guilt. Physical hunger has no guilt attached to it because you know you ate in order to maintain energy.

5.   Emotional hunger results from some emotional trigger. Physical hunger results from a biological need.

The Real Reason You're So Hungry – Imaginary Hunger

Did your answers to the five questions above reveal that you might be an emotional eater? Did you discover that you've been confusing emotional hunger with real, biological hunger? If so, the first question becomes – why?

The best way to explain what's going on is to consider that when you eat when you aren't really hungry, it's because you have two stomachs – one is real, the other imaginary. The hunger in your stomach is a signal to your brain that you need to re-fuel. It occurs when your system has a biological requirement for food. If that was the only signal of hunger you received, you'd be healthily slim. It's the imaginary stomach that causes the problems. The imaginary stomach sends out a signal demanding food as a result of complex and possibly negative emotions and unsolved problems. This is the moment when your stress and personal issues begin to assert themselves and you feel compelled to eat. Or, more accurately, to stuff yourself and anaesthetise the feelings of discomfort. Imaginary hunger exerts such a powerful influence that it compels you to eat almost anything to satisfy it.

There are certainly moments when each of doesn't really know what to do with ourselves. It can happen after work, when we are alone, late at night or even over the weekend. Does that sound familiar or do you have other triggers that compel you to sidle over to the fridge? All emotional eaters have specific issues that they want to avoid and, when those issues arise, the imaginary tummy howls with insistent urgency and you suddenly find yourself possessed by an out of control urge to eat.

FIGHTING FIBROMYALGIA With THE ANTI- INFLAMMATORY DIET By Mercedes Del Rey

BY THE SAME PUBLISHER

The Budget Paleo-Keto Holiday Delights

By Bestselling Author

Beran PARRY

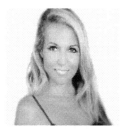

Eliminate the unnecessary, expensive food items and save big bucks on every shopping trip.
Get a healthier, fitter, trimmer and leaner body by eating smart on a budget because your health is truly priceless.

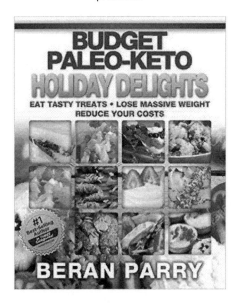

Please search the page below to get this book

www.amazon.com/gp/product/B017U69MOQ?ie=UTF8&camp=1789&creativeASIN=B017U69MOQ&linkCode=xm2&tag=onelifeblog-20

By Bestselling Author

Beran PARRY

The Paleo-Keto Post Holiday Detox

The tastiest way to flush out the toxins and eliminate those unwanted rolls of fat.
Celebrate the festive season with a revolution in your health, your waist size and your enjoyment. Because your health is the greatest gift you can give yourself.

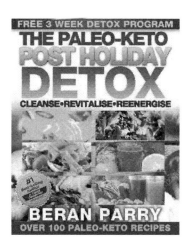

Please search the page below to get this book

www.amazon.com/gp/product/B017Z8Z36U?ie=UTF8&camp=1789&creativeASIN=B017Z8Z36U&linkCode=xm2&tag=onelifeblog-20

FIGHTING FIBROMYALGIA With THE ANTI- INFLAMMATORY DIET By Mercedes Del Rey

The most delicious way to eat your way to a leaner, fitter, healthier body and enjoy every single mouthful.

A deliciously enjoyable companion volume to Beran Parry's ground-breaking works on using the well-researched Paleo approach to the nutritional needs of modern, twenty-first century people in every part of the world. Full of the most deliciously nutritious recipes, this is an extremely useful guide to daily meal-planning throughout the year and adds variety and choice to please every taste and palate.

The PALEO Epigenetic RECIPE BOOK

420 Paleo Meals, 365 Paleo Recipes, 12 Paleo Food Categories

BONUS 12 WEEK PALEO DIET and MEAL PLANNER:

Your Ultimate Paleo Smart Genetic Guide

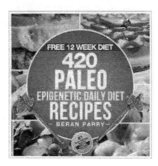

Please search the page below

www.amazon.com/gp/product/B00V8F9IFO?ie=UTF8&camp=1789&creativeASIN=B00V8F9IFO&linkCode=xm2&tag=onelifeblog-20

FIGHTING FIBROMYALGIA With THE ANTI- INFLAMMATORY DIET By Mercedes Del Rey

The Paleo Epigenetic Diet Bible is your new friend and helper, your constant companion and guide on the pathway to total wellness. It begins right here. With the most incredible selection of Paleo Diet Recipes ever!

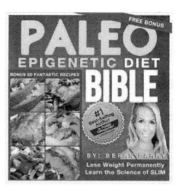

Search the page below for more information

www.amazon.com/gp/product/B00WKWZTQG?ie=UTF8&camp=1789&creativeASIN=B00WKWZTQG&linkCode=xm2&tag=onelifeblog-20

BERAN PARRY

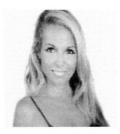

Please search over the internet

www.amazon.com/Beran-Parry/e/B00PSXHY4O/ref=ntt_dp_epwbk_0

Made in the USA
Middletown, DE
25 October 2018